Understanding the Patient's Perspective:

A Tool For Improving Performance

Joint Commission Mission
The mission of the Joint Commission on Accreditation of
Healthcare Organizations is to improve the quality of care
provided to the public.

ISBN: 0-86688-430-0

Library of Congress Catalog Number: 94-72831

Contents

Foreword

What do patients want? What do patients need? It is hard to imagine answering these questions without *asking* our patients. Yet in health care we have done just that for many years. Both clinicians and managers have done their best to meet patients' needs without systematically listening to the patients' perspectives on what they expect and need and how well, in the patients' judgment, those expectations and needs have been met. In essence, we have attempted to hit a target while blindfolded.

Increasingly, health care organizations are learning to take the blindfold off. To draw an analogy to manufacturing and service organizations that have adopted the principles of continuous improvement, in health care we are learning to listen to the "voice of the customer."

This book describes a framework for systematically learning about patients' needs and expectations, and their satisfaction with how well they are met, and using this information to continuously improve performance. It tells stories of some organizations that have learned how to listen to patients, and how these organizations were able to use their patients' perceptions to improve performance.

"The customer is always right." We've all heard it—even if most of us feel we have never actually experienced it as a customer. Does it apply to health care? Not exactly. This may be the reason that many clinicians, especially physicians and nurses, are uncomfortable equating "patient" with "customer." We know that scientific knowledge, technical experience, and skill are also critical components in the quality of health care and its outcomes. Sometimes the physician (or nurse, or social worker) does know best, and as patients, we expect them to deliver their best professional advice. So a framework for using patients' expectations, needs, and perceptions in an organization's improvement activities must merge these with other information—for example, about the environment, the state of the art, outcomes achieved, and the performance of other organizations.

The cycle discussed in Chapter 2 describes the need to *design* work processes—both clinical and nonclinical—upfront, using information about customers' needs and expectations, up-to-date knowledge, and the processes used by other organizations, as well as the outcomes they achieve. For clinical processes, the "customers" are patients. Up-to-date knowledge comes from the scientific literature and clinical practice guidelines, and information about other organizations comes from reference databases and benchmarking. Once a work process is in place, it is necessary to *measure* its performance, including measurements of outcomes (that is, the patients' health outcomes) and the processes used to achieve them, patient satisfaction, and costs. But measurements are only data. These data need to be *assessed*—transformed into information that can be used to answer the question, "Where can we improve?" and to decide which improvement opportunities should be priorities.

This assessment process makes use of statistical analysis tools, such as run charts, and process analysis tools, such as flowcharts. In addition, assessment is often dependent on comparisons—with the organization's own past performance, of other organizations recorded in reference databases, and current knowledge. Priority setting depends on knowledge of patient's priorities for improvement, resources needed, and criteria that include the frequency, impact (that is, risk), and cost of the process to be improved. Finally, a systematic process to *improve*, such as the Plan-Do-Check-Act cycle of Shewhart and Deming, can be used to redesign current processes to improve them or design new processes that lead to innovation. Patient' needs and expectations, and their satisfaction with current processes and their results, are used in the redesign of old processes and in the design of new processes—coming full circle in the cycle.

This may sound logical as *theory*, but does it work in *practice*? That is what this book is about—the transition from theory to practice in using patients' perceptions to improve organizational performance. Listening to our patients is not only key to their diagnosis and treatment, but to our organizations' performance as well.

Paul M. Schyve, MD
Senior Vice President
Joint Commission

Chapter 1

Examining the Patient's Perspective

Alice feels a lump in her breast. Maybe there is some pain with it; maybe there is no pain at all. All she wants is to have this lump go away. She lives with fear and uncertainty. "What's going on? What's wrong with me?"

Once Alice finds out she has breast cancer, she must deal with all sorts of issues. She's not the only one affected; her whole family must face this problem. "Yesterday I was feeling fine. Yesterday I didn't have this lump in my breast, or I didn't know I had it. Today, I'm sick. Today, I'm different."

The only time Alice had ever been in a hospital was to deliver her two daughters. Now, she feels as though she spends half her life in a wheelchair being pushed by people in white coats. She works full-time and takes care of a family. Now she must let others take control. "I feel like everyone is staring at me." She is asked to decide among a lumpectomy, mastectomy, radiation, chemotherapy, or chomoxifin—words she doesn't feel she fully understands and never connected with herself until today.

After her mastectomy, Alice finds it difficult to sleep. She is troubled by issues of self-image. "I was a mother and wife. Who am I now?" And the recovery—"Are these symptoms normal? Is the cancer coming back?"[1]

This example shows a patient's perceptions from the decision to seek care through diagnosis, treatment, discharge, and follow-up. These perceptions provide valuable information that, if solicited and appropriately used, could lead to improved performance of a health care organization. However, too often this type of patient input is not used to design the systems and processes of health care organizations. In many ways, the current health care systems have been developed around the needs of those who built and operated them, rather than the patients who are the most profoundly affected by the systems. For instance, most admitting and outpatient registration processes were developed to meet the needs of the admitting department, business office, medical record department, and discharge-planning staff, rather than patients.[2]

To begin improving health care systems so they better respond to patient input, it is necessary to see the organization through patients' eyes. This is done by collecting information about patients' needs, expectations, and satisfaction with services. That information can then be translated into design characteristics for specific processes. Then organizations can determine how well new or redesigned processes satisfy patients.

Traditionally, health care organizations have attempted to understand the patient's viewpoint through satisfaction surveys. Most hospitals score high on these surveys—often as high as 90% approval rating.[3,4] Yet, health care organizations must examine whether they are actually achieving the levels of patient satisfaction they think they are. Nelson and Niederberger report "a considerable gap between the content of many patient satisfaction surveys and what prior research has indicated to be important determinants of patient satisfaction."[5]

Patients and Joint Commission Standards

Many significant changes were made to the 1995 *Accreditation Manual for Hospitals* (*AMH*). One of the most significant is that it now traces the patient's pathway through the organization. By reorganizing the manual according to the important functions an organization provides (such as assessment of patients, rather than by departments or other structures), the Joint Commission is helping shift the focus back to the fundamental purpose for which a health care organization exists—to provide care to the patient.

Another important recent change in Joint Commission standards is the requirement to collect data about the needs and expectations of patients and others, as well as data about the degree to which these needs and expectations are satisfied. Table 1-1, page 12, lists the standards in the *AMH* that pertain to gathering and using patient input.

Although patients are unable to assess certain technical aspects of care (for example, whether a catheter is inserted appropriately), there are other aspects of care for which the patient can be the only judge (for example, whether he or she understood the physician's instructions). The Joint Commission standards recognize that organizations must gather patient input (among other data) to have complete information about organizational performance.

Purpose of this Book

Of course, it is not enough to simply gather patient input. Organizations must use that information to improve performance. This book is intended to help health care professionals in that effort.

Although this book provides a brief overview of methods for obtaining patient input, it is not a book about developing a sur-

Table 1-1. Standards in the 1995 *AMH* Related to Using Patient Input in Performance-Improvement Activities

"Leadership" Chapter

LD.1.3.3 [The plan(s) includes patient care services in response to identified patient needs and is consistent with the organization's mission.] Services are designed to be responsive to the needs and expectations of patients and/or their families/decision makers.

LD.1.3.3.1 The organization gathers, assesses, and takes appropriate action on information that relates to the patient's satisfaction with the services provided.

"Improving Organizational Performance" Chapter

PI.2.1.2 [New processes are designed well. The design is based on] the needs and expectations of patients, staff, and others;

PI.3 The organization has a systematic process in place to collect data needed to

- design and assess new processes;
- assess the dimensions of performance relevant to functions, processes, and outcomes;
- measure the level of performance and stability of important existing processes;
- identify areas for possible improvement of existing processes; and
- determine whether changes improved the processes.

PI.3.3.1 [The organization collects data about] the needs and expectations of patients and others and the degree to which these needs and expectations have been met; and

PI.3.3.1.1 These data relate to the relevant dimensions of performance.

---

vey instrument, holding a focus group, or conducting any other type of survey research. Many resources discuss those subjects in great depth (several are listed in Appendix B, pages 123–126). The purpose of this book is to provide quality improvement staff, organization leaders, and management with an understanding of how patient input can be used in performance-improvement activities. This chapter provides some background on the importance and types of patient input; Chapter 2 shows how that input can be incorporated in a cycle for improving performance; and Chapter 3 offers four examples of how health care organizations have used patient input to improve performance. Appendixes provide the Joint Commission's "Improving Organizational Performance" standards, further resources on using patient input, and examples of patient survey tools.

Background

Concern for the patient's viewpoint is intensifying in health care. Reiser proposes that the current focus on the patient can be traced to two recent movements—the medical ethics and medical outcomes movements.[6] Both of these have challenged the traditional view of medicine—that objective measures of a patient's illness are more reliable than the patient's own reports of how he or she felt. What has emerged instead is a more subjective perspective on illness. As Bartholome writes, "Patients not only have diseases but also experience them, as well as their effects. . ."[7]

The outcomes movement actually got its start at the turn of the century when EA Codman, MD, encouraged physicians to track the results of medical interventions. However, his ideas did not come to fruition until the 1980s when concern arose about rising costs and variation in physician practices. The patient's view is now playing an increasing role in the outcomes debate. A group involved in outcomes measurement recently determined that "the best criteria of whether the treatment succeeded" is "how the patient felt and functioned after therapy and whether the patient could return to work and normal social activities."[5]

Patient input has also become critical in the realm of medical ethics. The development of innovative technology and procedures as well as concern about costs have raised such questions as "What is a desired health outcome?" "When does life end?" "Who should decide?" As Reiser writes, "Who could weigh better the trade-offs of benefits and harms to self in relation to the goals, values, and obligations of life than the subject of an experimental intervention?"[6] After learning about what the patient values and finds important, clinicians can make better judgments about the technical aspects of care.

Other events and trends are also increasing patient involvement in health care. Patients themselves want to be more involved in the care process as they grow more sophisticated and educated about health issues. Moloney and Paul point out, "Baby Boomers who are caring for parents and aging themselves demand more information, involvement, control, and choice regarding the services they buy."[8] The release of comparative information on institutions and practitioners is also helping change the role of the patient. Patients, as well as purchasers, can now make more informed choices among providers.

Patient Needs and Expectations

Health care organizations must go beyond patient satisfaction surveys to gather patient input. To design processes that reflect patient input, organizations must learn patients' *needs and expectations*.

When a couple walks into a restaurant for dinner, they have needs and expectations in terms of both the product and service. For example, they need a meal and expect it will be served at the appropriate temperature within a reasonable period of time. They also need a server to take their order and perhaps to explain items on the menu. They expect that person to be knowledgeable, helpful, prompt, and courteous. Whether their needs and expectations are met for both the product and service may influence their overall satisfaction with the restaurant.

These same product/service needs and expectations exist when a patient is admitted to a health care setting. Those needs and expectations are much more difficult to discern, however, because of the complicated relationship that exists between patients and health care organizations . It is fairly easy for a person to describe what he/she expects from a meal in a restaurant (for example, the meal satisfies his/her hunger and tastes the way that it is expected). But it is more difficult for that same person to know what to expect after a heart valve replacement. The product being sought from a health care organization is a "technical" service, addressing an illness or health condition. This makes determining needs and expectations difficult because the patient does not always know what the long-term outcome should be or what he/she can expect in terms of health status. At times the patient may not even know he/she has a need (for example, he/she may not know his/her blood pressure is elevated).

The patient/health care organization relationship becomes even more complicated because the patient is having the service done to him/her. Metaphorically, it is as though a car drove itself into the car repair shop to be fixed. Thus, the patient's condition or illness may influence his/her perception of the care and caring provided.

Because of this complex relationship, a number of factors may limit the usefulness of patient input:

- Patients cannot accurately assess the technical competence of medical personnel. Furthermore, patients' physical or emotional status can easily impair judgment.
- Patients are influenced by nonmedical factors such as the interpersonal skills of the provider or the abundance (or lack) of sophisticated equipment.
- Patients are often reluctant to disclose what they really think because of their sense of dependency, fear, or prior failures in patient-physician communication.
- Patients cannot accurately recall aspects of the delivery process.[9]

Organizations should be aware of these issues as they develop appropriate questions to ask patients. They should also consider measures to lessen the impact of these factors when seeking patient input (for example, consider what time is best to interview a patient).

Types of Needs and Expectations

A patient has needs and expectations in relation to the *care* provided (or technical/product needs) and to the *caring* provided (or service needs). The amount of input patients can provide about these two different types of needs and expectations varies. Harper Petersen explains that "patients and caregivers are co-researchers, actively involved in discussing the patients' expectations and reactions to the quality of their care."[10] Staff members might begin by determining what the patient values, knows, and does not know about both the care and caring provided.

66*Several researchers have also tried to find ways to help patients overcome the 'passive patient' role and to become more knowledgeable and active participants in their own care. . . . [Researchers] studied the effects of giving patients with peptic ulcer disease short sessions, prior to each visit with the doctor, to review their medical record and encourage them to use the information to negotiate medical decisions. They found that patients provided with such sessions were twice as effective in eliciting information from their physicians and reported significantly fewer functional limitations as a result of their disease, when compared with a control group not given the sessions.*99

—from Kimberly D. Allshouse: Treating patients as individuals. In Gerteis M: *Through the Patient's Eyes*. San Francisco: Jossey-Bass Publishers, 1993, p32.

Care

The care provided includes both the clinical care (for example, an invasive procedure) and the supporting care (for example, patient education, nutrition services). Patients' view of the clinical care provided has become more central in measuring medical outcomes and health status since the emergence of the medical outcomes movement. Determining quality care "no longer rest[s] exclusively on traditional physiological and clinical indexes of how various body organs respond to treatment but will entail determining the effects of various treatments on the quality of patients' lives."[8] A team headed by John Ware, an expert in patient satisfaction, it has done a lot of work in this area; it has developed methods for classifying and translating patients' statements about how well they function and feel into objective measurements.[11-13]

Increasing patient satisfaction with medical outcomes/health status can be complicated because patients often have confused or unrealistic expectations. Many patients do not know what to expect in terms of how they will feel after surgery. Or, they might have unrealistic expectations and think they will be able to return to work in a week. Staff members first must learn what patients know and do not know and then determine what the patient should know about the clinical care being provided and the probable outcomes. This involves educating patients so their expectations are realistic and providing them with accurate information about their needs. This also makes the patient a better partner in the treatment process.

The patient's values and what he/she considers important to a quality life also affects satisfaction with medical outcome/health status. By involving patients in care decisions and helping them choose options that best meet their lifestyles and values, patients are more satisfied with the eventual outcomes. For example, Wennberg et al found that, for conditions such as an enlarged prostate or breast cancer, treatment decisions can only be made by first discovering the "patient's unique perceptions and valuations of the likely risks and benefits of alternative therapies." These researchers are developing interactive video disks, which use scripts and graphics to convey the nature of an illness and the effects of alternative treatments options from the patient's perspective.[14]

Attempts to increase satisfaction with those functions that support care (for example, admissions, patient education, family relations, nutrition services) can also be linked to determining what a patient knows and values. For example, some patients may be unfamiliar with the daily routine of a hospital. Because of this, they might have inaccurate expectations about meals, roommates, and so forth, and need to be educated. Patients' values also influence their satisfaction with the care given. For example, most patients consult their family when making treatment decisions. Thus, health care organizations might consider inviting patients' families to be present when discussing treatment options.

Caring

The caring provided, such as the interactions between the clinician and patient, is often referred to as the "art of medicine." Dr Herrman Blumgart defined the art of medicine as the "skillful application of scientific knowledge to a particular person for the maintenance of health or the amelioration of disease."[15]

The caring and respect given to the patient can influence health outcomes in many ways. According to Press et al, "Care is provided via interaction with

David Gustafson, PhD, admitted himself for open heart surgery and cardiac catheterization at the University of Wisconsin Hospitals. He went through the process from start to finish, except he wouldn't let surgeons cut him. He laid in bed for four hours with his legs straight to make sure bleeding stopped after the catheterization, he was wheeled around in a wheelchair, etc, looking for opportunities for improvement.

—from a seminar by
David Gustafson

individuals. Patient response to these interactions *plus* their experience with surroundings, amenities, and equipment have direct impact upon their understanding of the procedures, upon trust and compliance, upon stress levels, and thus—logically—upon the medical outcome itself."[16]

For instance, a lack of caring and respect can cause communication problems between patients and providers. As communication fails, the ability of professionals to effectively diagnose and treat patients tends to diminish sharply. Consider, for example, postoperative pain management. The communication of pain is a social transaction between caregiver and patient and, according to one source, the "single most reliable indicator of the existence and intensity of acute pain."[17] Successful assessment and control of postoperative pain depends in part on establishing a positive relationship between health care providers, patients, and, when appropriate, patients' families.

Again, health care organizations can begin to increase satisfaction with the caring provided by determining what patients know and value. Studies have already shown that patients consider the respect and caring they receive to be very important. One study found that patients typically focus on the physician's personality and interpersonal skills as measures of quality—that is, "the amount of time doctors spend with a patient, how much interest they show in who the patient is and in his or her well-being, how much information they provide, and whether they are compassionate and understanding."[18]

Recognizing the importance patients place on respect and caring, many health care organizations are placing a larger emphasis on interpersonal skills. Medical and other professional schools are requiring students to practice the art of medicine as well as the science. Some organizations are also designing new systems that can provide a high level of caring in innovative ways. For example, as a result of a needs assessment of breast cancer patients, the University of Wisconsin Hospital provides each breast cancer patient with a computer on discharge. In this way, patients can access information about breast cancer and communicate through e-mail with other patients any time of day or night (see Chapter 3 for more details on this example).

Three Levels of Expectation

Looking at different levels of expectations can help a health care organization determine where to place its priorities. Dr Noriaki Kano, one of the most prominent figures in Japan's quality movement, discerned three basic levels of customer reactions to quality features or characteristics. These three levels are referred to here as take-it-for-granted, expected, and exciting attributes.[19] Figure 1-1, page 21, illustrates the effect each of these has on patient satisfaction.

Take-it-for-granted attributes

Examples of attributes that patients "take for granted" in a health care organization may include matters such as physician skill, availability of technology and equipment, and systems set up so tests are not misplaced. Every new car purchaser assumes his/her car will have good brakes. Similarly, patients expect hospitals to provide skilled physicians and may assume that medical skill is relatively the same across hospitals. A patient may not respond favorably when a health care organization provides a competent service, but if the organization *fails to provide it* (for example, loses a patient's blood test), the patient will probably become frustrated or angry. Ensuring that take-it-for-granted features are present is considered by some to be the role of quality assurance. [20]

Expected attributes

Attributes that patients expect may include attention and concern shown by nurses and the accommodation of visitors. Like take-it-for-granted attributes, patients expect these characteristics to be

Figure 1-1. Levels of Patient Expectations

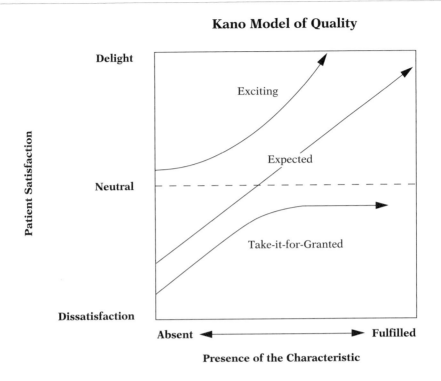

Kano Model of Quality

Figure 1-1. *As shown, the presence of a take it for granted characteristic will only leave patients feeling neutral. Organizations have the opportunity to delight patients with "expected" or "exciting" characteristics.*

SOURCE: *Based on Kano SN, et al:* Attractive Quality and Must-Be Quality. *Methuen, MA: GOAL-QPC, 1984. Used with permission.*

present, but that expectation is not assumed to the same degree that, for example, appropriate equipment may be. By providing expected attributes, an organization will help ensure that a patient's conscious desires for care and service are satisfied.

Exciting attributes

Patients may not expect exciting attributes, but are delighted when they are present. Examples of exciting attributes could include no paperwork on admission, extra time with a physician, or special concern from a nurse. The more useful yet unexpected a feature, the more likely it is to create true delight.

Meeting patient needs and expectations is like trying to hit a moving target. Something that was an exciting attribute ten years ago may be a take-it-for-granted attribute today. That is one reason it is important for health care organizations to keep a constant tab on patients' needs and expectations.

Determining What to Measure

A health care organization must prioritize what is important to know and measure in relation to patients' needs and expectations. Each patient arrives with varying degrees of conscious and unconscious needs and expectations. In setting priorities for gathering patient input, a health care organization should return to the fundamental need it fulfills in the community— providing care and services to patients. As the following studies show, organizations should focus first on improving those processes and services that affect patient health outcomes.

A study of 70,000 inpatients at Hospital Corporation of America looked at what caused a good or bad surprise for patients during their hospital stays. A good surprise was defined as something that surpassed patient expectations while a bad surprise failed to meet patient expectations. Extras and perks, or exciting attributes, that patients received were associated only with good surprises whereas expected attributes (such as attention and caring from nurses) caused both good and bad surprises. Aspects of care identified as take-it-for-granted either did not cause a surprise (for example, skill of physicians) or caused a bad surprise (for example, value/cost of care). From their findings, the researchers were able to show that a bad surprise reduces patient satisfaction (by -0.09) more than a good surprise increases it (by +0.03).[21]

These findings correlate with a study done of service industries such as car repair and life insurance. Researchers categorized customer expectations into five overall dimensions: reliability, tangibles, responsiveness, assurance, and empathy. Reliability is largely concerned with the service outcome (for example, the clinical care provided in a health setting), whereas the four other dimensions are more concerned with the service process (that is, the caring provided). The study concluded that "reliability is the most important dimension in meeting customer expectations." They also found that customers have a lower zone of tolerance for an unreliable service than for unresponsive or unempathetic service.[22]

These findings suggest that any exciting attributes offered the patient will ring hollow if the fundamental care they expected to receive is less than satisfactory. It goes back to the fundamental need the health care organization fulfills. Patients never forget why they were admitted to a hospital. Yet, in the 1980s, many organizations attempted to become more patient oriented by improving foodservice and other hotel-type services.

> **"**Xerox is hiring anthropologists to go into foreign society and learn how people work and xerox documents in their work environment.**"**
>
> —from a seminar given
> Eugene C. Nelson, DSc, MPH

When setting priorities for improvement, health care organizations should weigh what will have the greatest impact on patient outcomes. Although improving the delivery of meals might have some impact on patient outcomes (that is, reduce patient stress that might inhibit recovery), it is minimal when compared to the impact of such processes as patient assessment or patient education. As Nelson concludes ". . . it would be wise for most hospitals to continually improve their performance in the take-it-for-granted and expected areas. The superior hospital might go further by first identifying areas of exciting quality and then redesigning its internal processes so that patients' expectations can be surpassed consistently."[21]

Patient Input and Quality Improvement

Attention to the patient's perspective corresponds to the principles of quality improvement (also called "continuous quality improvement" and "total quality management") that are gaining widespread acceptance in health care today. The focus on the patient's viewpoint reflects the emphasis on the customer that is central to the theories of such quality improvement experts as W. Edwards Deming and Joseph Juran.

At the core of these theories is the concept that an organization is composed of processes, and to design effective processes, attention must be paid to each process's *customers* and *suppliers*. One crucial customer to many processes in a health care organization is the patient. As discussed in other Joint Commission publications,* organizations committed to quality improvement try to meet or exceed the needs and expectations of external customers (such as patients and their families) as well as internal customers (such as physicians and staff).

Recent studies show that organizations that focus improvement efforts around the needs and expectations of external customers, such as patients, are generally more successful. A study in the *The Economist* reports that two thirds of the companies that adopted quality improvement five years ago have since dropped it, calling it a waste of time and investment. However, the other third are convinced that quality improvement has

---

* Joint Commission publications on improvement theories and practice include *Framework for Improving Performance: From Principles to Practice*; *The Measurement Mandate: On the Road to Performance Improvement in Health Care*; *Exploring Quality Improvement Principles: A Hospital Leader's Guide*; and *Implementing Quality Improvement: A Hospital Leader's Guide*. All are available from the Joint Commission.

helped turn their companies around. The differentiating factor between these two groups was a focus on the external customer.[23]A University of Wisconsin literature review of improvement studies in several countries supports this finding. Gustafson concluded that "internal efforts of trying to smooth processes that the customer wouldn't notice tended to end up as failures."[1]

The discussion and examples in this book focus on using input from just one external "customer"—patients. However, the strategies and tools provided are applicable to learning about other customer groups as well. Organizations must strike a balance in meeting the needs and expectations of all its customers.

Given the complex relationship that exists between the patient and clinician, the term "customer" might

> **❝** *Paris-based Club Mediteranee makes extensive studies of the attitudes and preferences of its customers, particularly of national and ethnic differences that may influence their perceptions of quality and personal interaction. Club Med's chefs des villages, or village managers, are expected to know the basic attitudes and preferences of different customer nationalities and to train staff to serve them in ways keyed to their needs.* **❞**
>
> —excerpted from Karl Albrecht: *The Only Thing that Matters.* MYC: Harper Business, 1992

be difficult for some clinicians to associate with patients. However, in view of the rising costs associated with health care and the fact that health care is a service delivery business, much can be learned from thinking about patients as customers. Like a customer who enters a restaurant, a patient arrives as a customer at the health care organization with a set of needs and expectations.

Next Step

The next step is to find a way to incorporate patient input into an organization's improvement activities—that is, to gather relevant patient input and to use that input to improve existing processes or to design new processes. Chapter 2 describes a cycle for improving performance and suggests how patient input can be part of each step of that cycle. Chapter 3 follows this discussion with real life examples of how four health care organizations have used patient input to improve their performance.

Methods for Listening to the Patient: An Interview with Doris Quinn, MSN, RN

Doris Quinn, MSN, RN, is the Director of Process Improvement at Vanderbilt University School of Nursing and Medical Center (Nashville, Tenn.). Her role is to facilitate the integration of continual improvement philosophy and techniques in the nursing school's strategic-planning effort. She also serves as a consultant to managers at Vanderbilt University Medical Center in design/redesign of systems for patient care. Prior to this position, she was Director of Customer Knowledge and Quality Improvement at Hospital Corporation of America. Quinn is presently a doctoral candidate at Vanderbilt University School of Public Policy specializing in policy development and program evaluation.

Interviewer: What are some initial steps management can take toward making their organization more customer-focused?

Quinn: First, you need to develop a method of listening to the voice of your customers, especially the key customers [that is, patients, physicians, employees, payers]. Surveys are being developed all over the country—find some that meet your needs. [Be mindful that surveys should have validity and reliability.] You won't save money with a home-made survey if the results are questionable.

Surveys should have some open-ended questions to allow free expression of concerns and delights. Once data are being collected, *everyone* should read the surveys, including the verbatim comments. Managers should not "interpret" the verbatim comments, but allow their staff to read the complaints or compliments from many patients, over several data collection time periods. There are themes that will emerge over time that may point the way to high-leverage improvement opportunities. Customer feedback should be examined for such themes, not just individual comments.

Letters of praise and complaints are also part of this "voice of the customer." The idea is to read the letter or listen to the patient and think about the process(es) that created a good or bad experience. It is easy to discount complaints since we feel the patient was ill, under stress, etc. This attitude will make us miss the most important cue—that some processes are not working well.

Listening to physicians as customers is very important and often poorly done. It is critical to have a methodology that listens to *all* the physician customers. Follow-up is important. All customers want to know something is being done to improve.

Employees are probably the least listened to of the organization's customers. If employees are surveyed, and a plan is put in place to address the processes/systems that are not functioning properly, morale can be greatly improved. This may, consequently, improve employee interaction with physicians and the patients.

Interviewer: What type of strategies can a hospital set up to ensure the organization is continually tuned in to the needs and expectations of patients and other customers?

Quinn: It is very important that data collection not be a one-time deal when something goes wrong. Patients' needs and expectations will change over time, and if the hospital is not keeping its finger on the patient's satisfaction pulse, they may find their patients going elsewhere for care.

This is not just good business sense but good health care. A hospital needs to know what happens to patients during and after their stay in order to improve itself and the care it provides. We know that improving quality means decreasing the cost of waste and rework. If data are collected over time, the hospital may be able to pick out trends and shifts in patient satisfaction.

An example occurred in a hospital that saw a marked decline in satisfaction at various times. They could not understand why there were more complaints and unhappy patients some of the time and not others. When they plotted the data over time, they found that the satisfaction scores corresponded to specific months. This hospital did not staff up for the "flu" season and, therefore, had to deal with the high census without enough staff. Just when the nurses' complaints were rather strong, the flu season would end, they had enough staff, and the satisfaction scores returned to a higher level. Without the data plotted over time, this valuable information would have been missed.

Interviewer: What are some specific methods for collecting data over time?

Quinn: Methods for collecting data over time vary. Some hospitals collect data in "waves." Twice a year, three months worth of discharged patients are sampled and some patients are mailed a questionnaire. Other hospitals have a questionnaire that is filled out before the patient leaves the building. Still others have phone surveys once a month on a smaller number of recent discharged patients. The method will depend on the need of the organization and how much money it can spend.

Less formal methods are also important. Hospitals that are serious about meeting customer needs and expectations will use everyone in the organization to collect data. Employees do this by listening to what the patients, physicians, and other employees are saying. An unhappy customer means a process is not working well. If all hospital employees know the importance of being customer-focused they will want to share the complaint or the positive remark with someone.

The hospital needs to have a structure in place to listen to these customers. For example, one hospital had a one-page "opportunity for improvement" sheet that could be used by anyone in the organization to communicate ideas, concerns, suggestions, and, most importantly, complaints that employees might have heard from their customers. The sheet was sent to the quality improvement "coach" who then shared it with the senior leaders at their next meeting. The leaders prioritized improvement opportunities and chartered improvement teams. All improvement sheets were kept for action (either immediate or future) and the person sending the sheet was immediately given feedback by the senior leaders.

Interviewer: Is there any other advice you would give organizations?

Quinn: The last strategy that will ensure that customers are being heard is to create a culture that allows employees to be innovative. Caregivers have many ideas for improving their work, and management must be open to listen. Front-line workers must constantly make excuses to patients and other customers when processes break down. I would be willing to bet that they have many ideas that management has yet to ask them about.

Interviewer: What resources does an organization need to commit to accomplish these objectives?

Quinn: The resources needed include (1) money for surveys that will meet the needs of the organization and either a researcher or a firm to administer the survey and perhaps perform data analysis; (2) someone designated to collect customer information [such as a QI coach, marketing director]; (3) time to review data, make decisions about priorities, respond to feedback, and charter improvement opportunities by individuals or teams; and

(4) a mechanism in place that will tie the voice of the customer to the voice of the process.

Listening to patients, their families, physicians, vendors, payers, employees, and so forth, should become a priority for all health care workers. But once they have heard, they must have a way of directing the information to management so that appropriate action can be taken. Management, in turn, must have a process in place for listening to the customers and being able to take action.

References

1. Based on Gustafson DH: *Customer Needs Assessment* (seminar given at the National Forum on Quality Improvement in Health Care), Orlando, FL, Dec 1992.

2. Jablonski R: Customer focus: The cornerstone of quality management. *Healthc Financ Manage* 46: 17–18, Nov 1992.

3. McMillan JR: Measuring consumer satisfaction to improve quality of care. *Health Progr* 68: 54–55, 76–80, Mar 1987.

4. Pascoe GC, Attkisson CC: The evaluation ranking scale: A new methodology for assessing satisfaction. *Eval Program Plann* 6(3–4): 335-347, 1983.

5. Nelson CW, Niederberger J: Patient satisfaction surveys: An opportunity for total quality improvement. *Hosp Health Serv Adm* 35(3): 409–427, Fall 1990.

6. Reiser SJ: The era of the patient: Using the experience of illness in shaping the missions of health care. *JAMA* 269: 1012–1017, Feb 1993.

7. Bartholome WG: A revolution in understanding: How ethics has transformed health care decision making. *QRB* 18: 6–11, Jan 1992.

8. Moloney TW, Paul B: The consumer movement takes hold in medical care. *Health Aff* 10: 269, Winter 1991.

9. Vuori H: Patient satisfaction—An attribute or indicator of the quality of care? *QRB* 13: 106–108, Mar 1987. As reported in Nelson CW, Niederberger J: Patient satisfaction surveys: An opportunity for total quality improvement. *Hosp Health Serv Adm* 35(3): 409–427, Fall 1990.

10. Harper Petersen MB: Using patient satisfaction data: An ongoing dialogue to solicit feedback. *QRB* 15: 168–171, Jun 1989.

11. Tarlov AR, et al: The medical outcomes study: An application of methods for monitoring the results of medical care. *JAMA* 262(7): 925–930, Aug 1989.

12. Stewart AL, et al: Functional status and well-being of patients with chronic conditions: Results from the medical outcomes study. *JAMA* 262: 907–913, Aug 1989.

13. Wells KB, et al: The functioning and well-being of depressed patients. *JAMA* 262: 914–919, Aug 1989.

14. Wennberg JE, et al: An assessment of prostatectomy for benign urinary tract obstruction: Geographic variations and the evaluation of medical care outcomes. *JAMA* 259(20): 3027–3030, May 1988.

15. Blumgart H: Medicine: The art and the science. In Reynolds R, Stone J (eds): *On Doctoring.* New York: Simon & Schuster, 1991, pp 105–118.

16. Press I et al: Patient satisfaction: Where does it fit in the quality picture? *Trustee* 21: 8–10, 21, Apr 1992.

17. U.S. Department of Health and Human Services, Public Health Service, Agency for Health Care Policy and Research: *Acute Pain Management: Operative or Medical Procedures and Trauma Clinical Practice Guideline,* AHCPR Pub No. 92–0032. Rockville, MD, 1992, 11.

18. Walker AJ: Results of the Medicare beneficiary and physician focus groups. In Lohr KN (ed): *Medicare: A Strategy for Quality Assurance, Volume II: Sources and Methods.* Washington, DC: National Academy Press, 1990, pp 45–46.

19. Kano SN, et al: *Attractive Quality and Must-Be Quality.* Methuen, MA: GOAL/QPC, 1984.

20. Gustafson DH, et al: Assessing the needs of breast cancer patients and their families. *Qual Manag Health Care* 2(1): 6–17, Fall 1993.

21. Nelson EC, Larson C: Patients' good and bad surprises: How do they relate to overall patient satisfaction? *QRB* 19: 89–94, Mar 1993.

22. Pasasuraman A, et al: Understanding customer expectations of service. *Sloan Manage Rev* 32(3): 39–48, Spring 1991.

23. The Cracks in Quality, *The Economist,* Apr 18, 1992, pp 67–68.

Chapter 2

Using Patient Input in a Cycle for Performance Improvement

To effectively use patient input to improve performance, an organization needs a systematic method for gathering that input, assessing the data gathered, and using the information to improve current processes and design new processes. Such a systematic method should include the stages in the Joint Commission's cycle for improving performance. These stages are reflected in the Joint Commission's "Improving Organizational Performance" standards PI.2, PI.3, PI.4, and PI.5 in the 1995 *AMH*.

A Cycle for Improving Performance

This cycle is a flexible, logical approach to improving performance. The cycle is not completely new; it synthesizes various proven approaches to improvement and provides a common language to discuss systematic improvement. The cycle can be used by a single work group, by an organization, or even by a network of organizations. It can be used for a process that affects just a few staff members and patients or for a process that affects an entire organization. It is possible to enter the cycle at any stage.

The major stages of the cycle—as illustrated in Figure 2-1, page 33—are as follows:

- Design;
- Measure;
- Assess; and
- Improve.

A brief explanation of each stage follows, with a discussion of how an organization can use this cycle to gather and use patient input.

Design

In this cycle, *design* means designing new processes. Although processes in health care organizations often grow by increments, with steps and substeps added as new circumstances are encountered, a process should be carefully designed to meet specific objectives, including patient needs and expectations.

The decision to design a new process is not made lightly. New processes should be chosen and designed with careful consideration of the following: the organization's mission, vision, and strategic plan; data about organizational activities relevant to the process; current knowledge about the process; and organizational resources. Another crucial consideration in any new process is the needs and expectations of the process's customers and suppliers, including patients. Effective collection and interpretation of patient input ensure that a new process can meet patient needs and expectations—even exceed them.

Measure

Measure means collecting valid, reliable data—especially data about how a process is performing. In today's environment, measurement is an especially pressing concern for all health

Figure 2-1. Cycle for Improving Performance

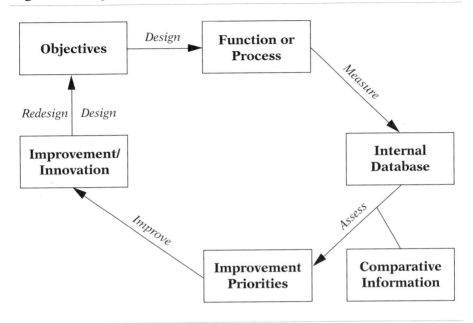

Figure 2-1. *This cycle offers a systematic method to improve functions and processes. The cycle is composed of activities (the lines and words above them) and inputs to and outputs from the activities (in boxes). This chapter explains how patient input can be incorporated into this improvement cycle.*

care professionals. The need to demonstrate effectiveness and efficiency requires organizations to quantify their performance with measures of patient health outcomes and resource use. And, of course, the desire and ability to meet community health needs require measuring those needs.

Measurement is important at several stages in the improvement process. Measurement about factors such as community health needs can help in new process design. Measurement about current processes can help demonstrate whether those processes are performing according to specifications or whether they require improvement. And measurement can help demonstrate whether an improvement action is having the desired result.

As discussed in Chapter 1, Joint Commission standards now require organizations to measure patient needs and expectations (as well as those of other important customers and suppliers). In addition, standards in the 1995 *AMH* ask that organizations collect data about

- outcomes;

- processes related to the important functions identified in the manual (for example, assessment of patients, care of patients, leadership, among others);

- high-volume, high-risk, and/or problem-prone processes; and

- processes related to use of surgical and other invasive procedures, use of medications, and use of blood and blood components and those for determining the appropriateness of admissions and continued hospitalization.

Assess

In this cycle, *assess* means translating data collected during measurement into information that can be used to improve performance. This assessment can take many different forms. Health care professionals assess data about community needs, organizational resources, and other factors before implementing a new process; they assess data about current performance to identify needs for improvement; they assess existing processes to understand how they are carried out; they assess the causes of current performance to help target actions for improvement; and they assess data about how a process performs after an improvement action has been taken.

Most assessment requires comparing data to a reference point. A reference point may be a historical pattern in the organization, the performance of other organizations as represented in aggregate external databases, external benchmarks, or practice guidelines. One possible point for comparison is the specifications an organization sets, based, in part, on patient input.

Certain kinds of assessment also require learning what factors cause current performance. This knowledge is gained by studying a process; identifying its steps and decision points; identifying the various people, actions, and equipment required for the process's outcome; finding links between variables in performance; and ranking the frequency of causes.

Intensive assessment of a process should result in identifying opportunities to improve root causes for its performance and should set priorities among those opportunities. The assessment can then identify root causes for its performance of processes chosen for improvement. Because improvement actions can lead to significant investment in time and effort, and can lead to significant improvement as well, organizations must consider their mission, strategic plans, resources, and other such issues when setting improvement priorities. One of the issues considered in setting priorities is the priorities of patients and other customers.

Improve

Improve means taking appropriate action based on measurement and assessment. Such action may involve redesigning an existing process or designing a new process to meet a defined objective (such as the needs and expectations of a patient group). Effective improvement actions involve the right people—those involved in and affected by a process, including patients. Improvement actions are carried out in a systematic manner and they are planned and tested before full implementation. Improvement actions must result in desired and sustained changes. When these actions involve changing an existing process shown to be problem prone, the actions must address root causes of the undesirable performance, rather than simply the most obvious manifestations.

Clearly, an important facet of improvement is careful measurement and assessment. When a new or redesigned process directly affects patients, that measurement and assessment must yield information about patients, including their own perceptions as well as their documented health status.

Using Patient Input in the Improvement Cycle

Although this book discusses using one source of information—patients—to improve performance, it is important to remember that organizations need to collect information from various sources, including other customers and suppliers, and weigh the disparate needs and expectations of different groups.

The following sections examine each stage of the improvement cycle—design, measure, assess, and improve—in terms of the patient. Chapter 3 then takes this discussion a step further by showing four specific examples of how these concepts have been enacted in health care organizations.

Design

Designing a process to use patient input in performance improvement requires reviewing

- the patient groups served by the organization;
- the important clinical and organizational functions that affect patients;
- the dimensions of performance that affect patients in each function; and
- the possible methods for gathering and using patient input.

The result should be a set of priorities for measuring patient input, along with a method for assessing the results and putting the information to use in improving organizational performance.

It is important to keep in mind that using patient input to improve performance is not an isolated activity. Rather, it should be linked—in the organization's strategic plan as well as in its practice—to organizationwide performance improvement.

For example, an effort to redesign the admission process would benefit from knowledge of patients' perceptions about the current process, as well as their expectations and perceived needs for the process.

Reviewing the Patient Groups Served

Each segment of the patient population has its own needs and expectations. Therefore, it is important to look at those various patient groups when determining how to effectively use patient input in performance improvement.

One way to segment patients would be by history: current patients, former patients, potential patients who go to a competitor, potential patients who choose different types of services to fulfill the same basic need, and so on. Another way to segment patients would be by diagnosis or illness, each of which carries distinct patient needs and expectations and can affect how patients perceive their health care experience.

A health care organization might want to further identify those patient groups that are important to its success as an organization. For example, a hospital might identify cardiac patients or obstetric patients as key customer segments if these patients are a large source of revenue or if the hospital wants to establish itself as a center of excellence in these areas. This idea reflects an organization's mission and vision as they pertain to fulfilling the community's health care needs and to being a financially viable organization.

Reviewing the Important Functions That Affect Patients

At the same time leaders are identifying key patient groups, they should identify those functions and processes that are most important to their operations. The Joint Commission has begun to identify those organizational functions that most powerfully affect patient outcomes, as well as key hospital structures that carry out important functions (see Table 2-1, page 39). In fact, the standards manuals are now organized according to these key functions. Health care organizations might use this list of functions as a starting point and add others that are specific to their organizations.

Thinking about patients in terms of the important functions that affect them helps an organization link patient input to the activities of the organization, and thus use that input to improve those activities.

Reviewing the Dimensions of Performance That Affect Patients

Each function carried out by a health care organization has more than one dimension of successful performance. Therefore, when considering how to gather patient input, it is important to identify not just the functions that affect various patient groups, but the dimensions of performance most important to patients and their perceptions.

The Joint Commission has identified nine dimensions of performance, which can help an organization determine how its functions may affect patients:

- Efficacy;
- Appropriateness;
- Availability;
- Effectiveness;
- Timeliness;
- Safety;
- Efficiency;
- Continuity; and
- Respect and Caring.

Table 2-1. Important Functions Identified in the 1995
Accreditation Manual for Hospitals

Patient-Focused Functions

- Patient Rights and Organizational Ethics

- Assessment of Patients

- Care of Patients

- Education

- Continuum of Care

Organizational Functions

- Improving Organizational Performance

- Leadership

- Management of the Environment of Care

- Management of Human Resources

- Management of Information

- Surveillance, Prevention, and Control of Infection

Structures with Functions

- Governance

- Management

- Medical Staff

- Nursing

Table 2-2, page 40, defines each of these dimensions. The relationships between patient groups, important functions, and dimensions of performance are illustrated in the "quality cube" shown in Figure 2-2, page 41.

Although all these dimensions of performance are undeniably important, patients may value some of these dimensions more highly than physicians or purchasers do. In addition, even when patients and others agree about the value a certain dimension

Table 2-2. Dimensions of Performance

- **Efficacy**—of the procedure or treatment in relation to the patient's condition. The degree to which the care/intervention for the patient has been shown to accomplish the desired/projected outcome(s).

- **Appropriateness**—of a specific test, procedure, or service to meet the patient's needs. The degree to which the care/intervention provided is relevant to the patient's clinical needs, given the current state of knowledge.

- **Availability**—of a needed test, procedure, treatment, or service to the patient who needs it. The degree to which appropriate care/intervention is available to meet the patient's needs.

- **Timeliness**—with which a needed, test, procedure, treatment, or service is provided to the patient. The degree to which the care/intervention is provided to the patient at the most beneficial or necessary time.

- **Effectiveness**—with which tests, procedures, treatments, and services are provided. The degree to which the care/intervention is provided in the correct manner, given the current state of knowledge, in order to achieve the desired/projected outcome for the patient.

- **Continuity**—of the services provided to the patient with respect to other services, practitioners, and providers and over time. The degree to which the care/intervention for the patient is coordinated among practitioners, among organizations, and across time.

- **Safety**—to the patient (and others) to whom the services are provided. The degree to which the risk of an intervention and risk in the care environment are reduced for the patient and others, including health care practitioners.

- **Efficiency**—with which services are provided. The relationship between the outcomes (results of care/intervention) and the resources used to deliver the care/intervention.

- **Respect and Caring**—with which services are provided. The degree to which the patient or a designee is involved in his/her own care decisions and to which those providing services do so with sensitivity and respect for the patient's needs, expectations, and individual differences.

Figure 2-2. The Quality Cube

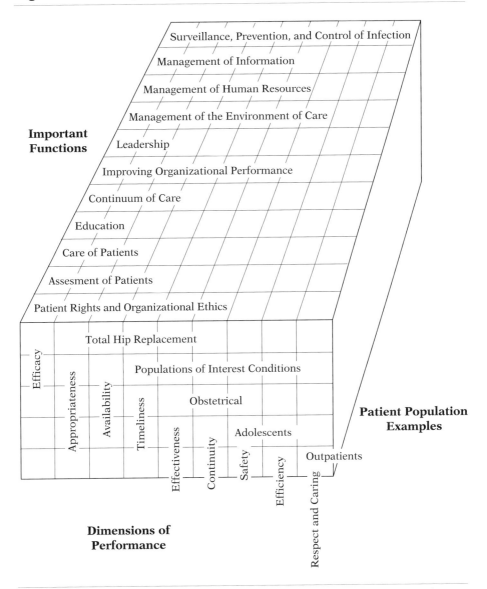

Figure 2-2. *This diagram illustrates the complex interactions among the various dimensions of performance, patient groups, and important functions of a health care organization.*

SOURCE: *This figure is based on the quality cube that appeared in* The Quality Letter for Healthcare Leaders, *May 1994, p 33.*

has, patients may define that dimension differently than another group. For example, physicians and patients would concur that assessments should be done on a timely basis; however, a physician's definition of timeliness and how much emphasis he/she places on this characteristic may very well differ from a patient's definition and emphasis. It is also important to note that in many instances, patients may have a limited ability to judge certain dimensions of performance (for example, the appropriateness of a certain procedure).

Different groups of patients may also place varying degrees of emphasis on a particular dimension. For example, trauma patients may place a higher emphasis on timeliness of assessment than obstetric patients would. It is these differences in emphasis that are important to discern when trying to use patient input in performance improvement.

Choosing Methods to Measure, Assess, and Improve

Considering the patient groups served, the functions that affect patients, and the dimensions of performance that patients value can help an organization decide what patient input to gather. However, before actually setting priorities for gathering patient input, an organization needs to consider how that data will be gathered, assessed, and used to improve the organization's overall performance through the design of new process or redesign of existing processes.

The methods to measure, assess, and improve processes using patient input should not be chosen in isolation. Rather, an organization should consider how best to integrate patient input into its current organizational improvement activities. Having said that, it is also important to note the methods and challenges unique to collecting patient input. The following sections of this chapter present more detail on how to measure patient needs and expectations, how to assess the data gathered, and how to use patient input to improve performance.

Setting Priorities for Gathering Patient Input

Like the methods for using patient input, the priorities for gathering patient input should not be identified in isolation. The priorities need to reflect the organization's mission, vision, and strategic plan; the organization's resources; and criteria such as the high-volume, high-risk, high-cost, or problem-prone nature of the patient groups or diagnoses being considered.

In addition, organization leaders should integrate priorities for patient input with other improvement priorities; indeed, most improvement activities an organization designates as high-priority would benefit from patient input.

In setting priorities, leaders need to select any types of patient input that need to be gathered on an ongoing basis. Such input would then be periodically assessed to determine whether an intensive improvement effort is warranted. That intensive effort would require more in-depth patient input and assessment of that input. Leaders may also select certain processes for intensive study without waiting for continuous measurement to trigger such an effort. Typically, such processes would be of very high priority for the organization because of their importance to the mission, their high volume, their problem-prone nature, their high cost, and so forth. When these processes affect patients directly—or even indirectly—understanding the patient's perspective is necessary.

Measure

The goal of measurement is to obtain valid, reliable data that can be translated into information about an organization's performance. Measuring patient needs, expectations, satisfaction, and other perceptions, therefore, requires a systematic method to ensure patient input is valid and reliable, and that it can be linked to organizational performance.

Any plan for measurement, including one for gathering patient input, should address the following:

- *What* data will be collected;
- *Who* will be involved in the collection; and
- *When, where,* and *how* the data will be collected.

Quinn offers this valuable list of questions that staff should answer in planning for data collection:

- *What data do we need?* What questions do we want answered? Are we interested only in exploring patient needs and expectations or do we want to test possible correlations and/or cause-and-effect relationships? What variables are we concerned with (for example, age of patient)?

- *Why do we need these data?* What are we going to do with the data? To whom are we going to give the data?

- *What data do we already have and what data do we need to obtain?* Do we have data sources currently available where some or all of this information can be obtained (for example, letters of complaint, organizationwide satisfaction surveys)? Are other departments/disciplines conducting similar studies? What additional data do we need?[1]

The form provided in Figure 2-3, pages 45 and 46, may help those involved in gathering patient input answer some key questions when planning the activities.

It is important to note that the measurement method varies depending on the process, patient group, diagnosis, or other subject being measured. Therefore, those involved in measurement must make sure they have a clear understanding of measurement's purpose and the limits of the subject being measured.

Seeking Expertise

Of course, measurement should not be undertaken without the necessary expertise in the tools and techniques. Gathering patient input has its own special challenges that a person with experience can help meet.

Figure 2-3. Sample Form for Planning to Gather Patient Input

Purpose of the Project

1. In a few sentences, describe the purpose of the effort to gather patient input.

2. Check the category(ies) that best describes the type of study you want to conduct:

    ____ *explorative study*. If an explorative study, what is it that you want to explore?

    ____ *correlations study*. If a correlations study, what correlations are you trying to establish? What variables are involved?

    ____ *causal-analysis study*. If a causal-analysis study, what causal relationships are you trying to establish?

3. Do you see this initial study leading to another? For example, if you are exploring patient needs, do you want to conduct a satisfaction survey at a later point?

What Information Do You Need?

4. List the questions that you want answered in this project.

    •

    •

    •

(continued on next page)

Figure 2-3. Continued

5.   How will the results of this project be used? Who will use these results?

6.   Are you aware of any current data sources available where some or all of the information you are seeking can be obtained (for example, letters of complaint, organization-wide satisfaction survey)? Are you aware of any other departments/disciplines conducting similar studies?

Design of the Project

7.   Define the population involved.

8.   Determine the sample you would like to use.

9.   Is there a particular method for gathering input you prefer to use (for example, focus group, survey)? If so, why?

Figure 2-3. *This form can be used to plan efforts to gather patient input that will later be used to improve performance. If seeking advice of a research expert, this form will provide much of the basic information the expert will need.*

There are a variety of places to find such expertise. Larger organizations might have marketing managers or departments, or they might hire outside marketing consultants to help them in this area. Many health care organizations committed to quality improvement are hiring or consulting with industrial engineers. Academic medical centers often have internal research departments staffed with experts in statistics and research methods. Even in small organizations, there may be pockets of this knowledge. For example, a social worker with a doctorate is usually trained in survey methods.

Before staff seek the assistance of a research expert, they should identify the questions they want the study to answer. The form in Figure 2-3 can help in this task.

Types of Measurement

Although this book does not examine in detail the means for gathering patient input, an overview of types of measurement that can be used should prove helpful.

Although there is no set formula for gathering patient input, organizations often begin with an *explorative* study of patient needs and expectations; then, they may conduct a *correlation* study to test possible relationships among variables; and finally they may undertake an even more detailed *causal-analysis* study of those relationships. The following sections briefly describe these types and the methods used to carry them out. Table 2-3, page 48, lists the most common methods used to gather patient input.

❝*David Kelley, whose company IDEO Product Development, Evanston, IL, "holds hundreds of patents," swears by direct observation as the key to innovation. Before designing a beach chair for a client, IDEO staff spent time observing people at the beach. "What we found was that as people sit on their chairs, they arrange themselves relative to the sun in a way that's comfortable," said Kelley. "But as time passes, the sun moves, so the people have to keep rearranging themselves." As a result of this research, IDEO invented a beach chair with a ball on the bottom so you can tilt and swivel and follow the sun.*❞

—Van J: No lone geniuses, today's inventors explore in teams. *Chicago Tribune*, Aug 15, 1993, Section 7, p 5.

Table 2-3. Methods for Obtaining Patient Input

The following are some popular methods for obtaining patient feedback. Some advantages and disadvantages of each method are listed. Readers interested in learning more about these methods will find some additional resources listed in Appendix B.

- **Focus groups.** A small group of patients (that is, eight to twelve people) is assembled and a moderator seeks their input concerning a particular issue(s).

- **Critical incident method.** An interviewer asks a patient to think about a specific event and describe the critical incidents that come to mind. (See page 77 in Chapter 3 for a example of this method.)

- **Direct observation.** Staff observe patients and make deductions about their needs and satisfaction. An alternative to this method is to go "undercover" as the patient.

- **Content analysis of letters and comments.** Staff assess letters that patients write or comments they share.

- **Written surveys.** These instruments are mailed or passed out to a sample of patients who then fill in their responses.

- **Archival studies.** In these studies, staff study patient effects for clues into their needs and wants. For example, they might observe the food patients leave on their trays to assess what food patients like and do not like.

- **Telephone surveys.** These are similar to written surveys except patients respond to questions over the phone.

- **Interviews.** Interviewers ask a sample of patients a series of questions either face-to-face or over the phone.

Explorative studies

As the term suggests, explorative studies help uncover what patients need, want, or feel is important. The purpose is to learn and add knowledge—not just confirm what is thought to be true. Staff need to approach explorative studies with an open mind. Techniques such as focus groups, face-to-face interviews, the critical incident method, or direct observation are typically used in explorative studies. These methods generally produce *qualitative data*, or data describing kinds and types of expectations, occurrences, conditions and so forth.

An explorative study is often the first phase of gathering patient input. For example, if a hospital wants to design an outpatient AIDS clinic, staff might begin by exploring what is important to AIDS patients, using methods such as focus groups, interviews, and direct observation. From these methods, the hospital might develop a list of overall needs and expectations that patients have regarding the outpatient clinic.

Correlation studies

Correlation studies are conducted to assess possible relationships among variables. Health care organizations might take the insight gleaned from explorative research and conduct a more structured study to determine if correlations exist.

In designing a correlation study, staff need to consider possible relationships in advance. For example, staff might suspect that the needs of AIDS patients vary according to age. They may also think that the manner in which patients contracted the disease affects their needs. If staff want to test for these variables, the survey instrument needs to ask respondents for this information. The sample also needs to include a representative number of patients in each category.

Correlation studies typically use methods such as mail surveys, phone surveys, and archival studies. These methods can provide *quantitative data*, or data expressed as numbers. However, most surveys use some open-ended questions that provide qualitative data to help guide interpretation.

Correlation studies suggest possible relationships, but they do not assert causality. Staff need to be careful not to draw causal relationships from correlation studies. This goes beyond the data. To determine if there may be a cause-and-effect relationship, staff must conduct a causal-analysis study.

Causal-analysis studies

Causal-analysis studies are more detailed examinations of causal relationships than can be determined through correlation studies. There are several different types of causal-analysis studies. One type studies a population before and after an intervention. For example, staff might discover through explorative research that families would like to be able to visit patients in the recovery room after surgery. Worried about the effect such a visitation policy would have on patients' health, nurses may decide to first test the policy on the cardiac intensive care unit. They then can compare patient satisfaction and health outcomes before and after the policy was instituted.

Needs Assessment

One term often applied to gathering patient input is "needs assessment." Generally, a needs assessment is an explorative study that helps health care providers understand what it is like to be a patient. For example, a needs assessment for hip replacement patients might ask patients whether it is best for them to receive pain medications before or after physical therapy. The purpose is *not* to determine whether patients were satisfied with the care provided, but to learn what is important to patients.

The ultimate goal of a needs assessment is to determine patients' "root want(s)." Patients often do not state their root wants at the outset, but those wants can be uncovered with skillful queries. For example, the comment "I would like more attention from nurses" could refer to several things—the number of nurses on the floor, the nurses' ability to respond to the call button, the amount of time nurses spend with patients, or the nature of the interaction between the nurse and patient. Follow-up questions can help determine which of these may be the root want.

Day writes, "If the questioning process does not aim at this root want, the value of the data suffers measurably. Once the interview is over and the customer has left, it is virtually impossible to determine what was meant by a comment that was not fully understood."[2]

As mentioned earlier, methods such as interviews, direct observation, and focus groups are useful in an explorative study (or needs assessment). Another useful method is the critical incident technique, which asks patients to think about a specific event and describe the important incidents that come to mind. This technique is discussed at length in Example 1 in Chapter 3, pages 77–82.

Indicators

Finally, when discussing measurement—including collecting patient input—it is important to address the concept of *indicators*.

An indicator can be defined as follows:

- A valid and reliable quantitative process or outcome measure related to one or more dimensions of performance such as effectiveness and appropriateness; and

- A statistical value that provides an indicator of the condition or direction over time of an organization's performance of a specified process, or an organization's achievement of a specified outcome.[3]

An indicator, then, is a key tool for measuring performance in any organization. Some indicators can be used to continuously measures certain processes (or outcomes related to a process), whereas a more detailed set of indicators may be used to measure performance as part of a specific improvement effort.

Some of the indicators that an organization continuously measures should address patient needs, expectations, and satisfaction. In addition, when more intensive measurement requires patient input, such indicators should be developed and pertinent data should be collected. The following is one example of an indicator that measures patient input (this indicator addresses the patient assessment process):

Patients state that physicians, nurses, and others allow adequate time for a clear and thorough discussion of their symptoms and needs.

The most common method for collecting data for such indicators is an organizationwide satisfaction survey. For each indicator, questions can be developed that measure patients' satisfaction in that area. For the above indicator, a survey might ask patients to rate (on a scale of 1 to 5) or report on (yes/no) whether caregivers allowed adequate time for discussion of their symptoms.

Several patient satisfaction surveys have been developed by other organizations that health care organizations can consider and adapt. (Appendix C, pages 127–151, contains examples of such surveys.) Furthermore, some organizations have developed patient satisfaction surveys that health care organizations can adopt as their own. Many of these organizations will also collect the survey data and provide analysis. One advantage of these surveys is that health care organizations can often compare their performance against other organizations. Typically, organizations are able to add organization-specific questions to these surveys.

Even if health care organizations decide to adopt predeveloped surveys, they should still hold focus groups, observe patients, and use other data-collection methods to gain first-hand knowledge about their patients' needs and expectations.

Developing a Patient Measurement System for the Future: An Interview with Eugene C. Nelson, DSc, MPH

Dr Nelson is the Director of Quality Education, Measurement and Research at the Dartmouth-Hitchcock Medical Center in Lebanon, NH, and Professor of Community and Family Medicine at Dartmouth Medical School in Hanover, NH. He has conducted extensive research on customer measurement within health care. This sidebar is excerpted from an interview with Dr Nelson, which appeared in the September 1993 issue of The Joint Commission Journal on Quality Improvement.

Interviewer: In developing a system to measure patient needs and satisfaction, what different types of measures should a hospital set up?

Nelson: There are two kinds of measures hospitals should consider: one involves understanding the goodness of the care experience from the patient's point of view (often called patient satisfaction); the other is to understand the outcomes of care from the patient's point of view (that is, health status/health outcomes).

Hospitals also need to consider the different levels of measures that are needed. A good way to understand this is to think of a tree. A tree begins at the trunk and spreads out into branches, then limbs, then twigs, and finally leaves. In designing a measurement system, it is often smart to start at the trunk—to get some overall measures of patient needs and satisfaction and to monitor the variation in care and the level of care from the patient's vantage point.

These "trunk like" measures provide bottom-line indicators of satisfaction. That's level one. At level two, you can start to get out to major branches of the tree that feed overall satisfaction and that feed overall outcomes.

Interviewer: At what level would you apply your resources?

Nelson: It is not an either/or process. Instead, it is a *both/and* process. Different people have different information needs. In designing a measurement system, you have to understand the different users and the different uses.

For example, the board of trustees is legally responsible for the care given to patients and needs to know about patient benefit. The chief executive officer of the hospital and the various senior people have a need to know about overall levels of quality. It is useful for leaders to have measures in place to understand the levels of quality, the variation, and so forth.

But, these overall measures are not very helpful for diagnosing where to make improvements or assessing if smaller improvements have been made. You've got to get out in the tree—the branches, the limbs, the leaves. You have to dig deeper to understand where the greatest zones for dissatisfaction are, what specific features and actions are actually stimulating the problem of dissatisfaction or creating the delight.

Interviewer: Aside from using patient feedback for identifying areas for improvement, how else do you see this feedback being used?

Nelson: Beside identifying problems, this information can be used to begin diagnosing the causes of a problem. You can start understanding the sources of variation, some of which are desired and some of which are undesired.

Let's take one area in which patients are often dissatisfied—the billing process. As staff flowchart this process and start to understand billing as a process with inputs, outputs, and outcomes, they begin to see how the process really works. At this point, staff can get the patient to report on each step of the process into which they have insight. Using focus groups and open-ended interviews, staff determine what the patient quality characteristics are of each step in the process, including the outcome.

Based on this information, staff might create a 30-item survey to gather ratings and reports of the billing system from the patient's point of view, as did the Hospital Corporation of America. This process allows hospitals to get very specific, fine-grained branch, limb, and sometimes even leaf information on the billing system as filtered through the eyes of the patient.

Interviewer: So, does it come down to an understanding of the PDCA [Plan-Do-Check-Act] cycle?

Nelson: In the background of what we're talking about is the concept of PDCA. But, in the foreground, we're connecting the process with the patient's view of the process. Ratings and reports of the patient's view provide baseline data for the "Plan" stage and follow-up data for the "Check" stage. Having a diagnosis from the patient of where the problems are in the process helps in the planning stages. This information helps in deciding what part or parts of the process to focus on.

Let's draw a simple flowchart of the care process: A patient has a medical need(s), accesses the system, and goes through admission and registration; data are collected on the patient, and the patient is assessed; a decision is made, treatment is given, and he or she goes through recovery, discharge, and follow-up to receive some health benefit.

You can look at the goodness of that core process from the point of view of the different customers. At each step, goodness can be defined from either the doctor's, nurse's or patient's point-of-view, and so forth. Essentially, you are applying different "lenses" to analyze the goodness of the process and the outcome.

Interviewer: To go back to trunk-level measures, how do you tie measures of patient needs and satisfaction with other measures that a hospital has in place [for example, financial data, utilization review]?

Nelson: Let's compare a hospital to another type of complicated system—the jet airplane. In the cockpit of this airplane, pilots can continually refer to an instrument panel that provides readings on the key aspects of flight [for example, altitude, direction, air pressure]. If the hospital system had a similar instrument panel, it would include a set of measures that related to the performance of the whole system.

To design this instrument panel, you need to identify key system performance measures. It helps to think of the basic aspects of the hospital system: inputs, processes, outputs, outcomes, customer judgements, community needs, plans to improve, and so on. At Dartmouth-Hitchcock Medical Center (DHMC), our system performance measures include indicators in most of these areas.

Patient-based measures may be part of your instrument panel, but they do not comprise the whole instrument panel. You need a multiplicity of measures to understand how different critical aspects of the hospital system are functioning.

Interviewer: Do all these measures on your instrument panel flow off your vision and goals?

Nelson: Yes. If you have a clear mission and vision, then the instrument panel helps you understand the extent to which you are attaining your mission and starting to realize your vision.

Interviewer: Looking five or so years in to the future, what do hospitals need to consider in designing a quality measurement system?

Nelson: More and more organizations are realizing that they will be successful to the extent that they can manage and improve the value of health care for those conditions for which patients come to them most frequently—whether it be pregnant patients, hip-replacement patients, cardiac patients, or oncology patients.

We'll start seeing what I call disease-specific or condition-specific "value compasses." On the compass, the four cardinal points might represent the following: clinical outcomes [mortality, morbidity, complications, and symptoms], general health status [physical, emotional, and social functioning], the patient's assessment of the goodness of care [patient satisfaction], and total cost, which includes direct medical costs [for example, hospital charges, drug costs] and indirect social costs [for example, time lost from work].

This compass provides a way of measuring the value of care provided to an individual patient or set of patients [value being the function of quality in relation to cost]. For example, a hospital could determine the value of care provided to the individual CABG [coronary artery bypass graft] patient or for the last 100 CABG patients. You could plot this information over time using a control chart to reveal variation or display aggregate measures for the last 100 patients. By "hanging" this value compass at the end of the core process, the clinical team will be able to assess the results of the process and start hanging measures of key process variables off the care process flowchart.

Interviewer: What else should hospitals consider?

Nelson: Another thing that is going to be increasingly common in the next five years is real-time assessment of critical processes and outcomes by the front-line providers [that is, physicians, therapists, nurses]. I think that we will see people getting more real-time feedback on critical processes, because there will be more knowledge of which processes really are critical.

Interviewer: What do you mean by "real time" measures?

Nelson: There can be real-time measures of both outcomes and processes. An outcome example might be a real-time measure of health status. For example, following a post-hip-replacement patient at two weeks, one month, three months, and six months. If you have real-time measures of outcomes when making a clinical assessment, you can see how the patient is doing and better match total regimen for the patient with total health need [biological, physical, and psychosocial functioning].

On the process side, let's take an example from Intermountain Health System [Salt Lake City]. Under the direction of Dr Brent James, they've identified very important variations in postsurgical deep wound infection rates. They traced these variations upstream and found that one major source was the timing of the prophylactic antibiotic [that is, the medication that prevents wound infections]. So Intermountain standardized the timing of the antiobiotic and built it into their care protocol so they know in "real-time" when this patient should get the antibiotic. The care team now gets real time prompts [for example, the 15-minute time segment when this patient should get the antibiotic].

Interviewer: Are there any examples of real-time prompts related to patient satisfaction?

Nelson: Sure, one area that is always problematic is the goodness of the communication process around the time of discharge. We just conducted a series of focus groups on CABG [coronary artery bypass graft] and PTCA [percutaneous Transluminal coronary angiography] patients, and this communication process was pinpointed as an area where we could improve. To develop real-time prompts in this area, we developed a checklist that included those critical issues patients or their families need to know about before being discharged. As part of the hospital discharge process, the patient or family member would need to complete the checksheet. Such a checklist would provide real-time feedback to help hospital staff to consistently meet informational needs before the patient goes home.

Assess

Raw data alone cannot be the basis for improving performance. Data collected about patient needs, expectations, satisfaction, and other matters must be carefully assessed. The assessment

- provides information about current performance;
- identifies opportunities for improvement;
- helps set priorities among the multiple opportunities; and
- helps identify root causes that can be addressed to bring about improvement.

This assessment can help an organization identify root causes of current performance, suggest actions that will improve current performance, and suggest specifications for new processes.

When patient input is gathered continuously, periodic assessment is necessary to determine whether more intensive measurement and assessment may be required. For a specific improvement project, assessment should lead to improvement actions.

Types of Assessment

Different types of measurement, and different subjects of measurement, require different types of assessment. For example, if measurement is designed to explore patients' needs and expectations, then assessment of the findings may focus on finding common themes. If, however, an organization is measuring to determine correlations or causal relationships, then assessment must identify those relationships. Assessment must look back to the original intent of the study (that is, do these data demonstrate what we thought they would?) and look forward to future studies (that is, what do these data *not* demonstrate? what else do we want to know?).

In particular, the approaches to assessment differ significantly when data are primarily qualitative (that is, categorical data) or quantitative (that is, data expressed as numbers).

Assessing Qualitative Data

Unlike quantitative data, assessing qualitative data does not necessarily require statistical expertise. It does, however, require a solid understanding of the process being studied and an ability to organize the patient input that has been gathered. One method used to assess qualitative data is called *content analysis*. Readers may be familiar with affinity diagrams, which work on the same principle.

A simple way to carry out content analysis is to divide the ideas patients express into separate content categories, placing each idea on a separate card. For example, one patient comment might be:

The nurses were very kind, but they were too busy
to respond quickly to my requests.

Staff might divide this comment onto two separate cards, one stating, "Nurses were very kind," and the other stating, "They [the nurses] were too busy to respond quickly to my requests."

Once all patient responses are placed on cards, the cards are sorted into meaningful categories. For example, the two cards above might fall under "Nurses' attitudes" and "Nurses' responses." Frequencies are then determined for each category. For example, one category might have 20 cards, another might have 40.

Such an assessment of qualitative data is an excellent opportunity for staff to listen to and understand the patient's voice.

Assessing Quantitative Data

Assessing quantitative data requires more advanced statistical knowledge. Many organizations hire outside companies to analyze these data. A number of computer software packages are also available that will perform such analyses. Users of software packages, however, must have a solid understanding of statistics.

Assessment of quantitative data often examines the variation in the process being measured. All processes have variation. *Special-cause variation* is the variation that results from causes outside the way a process is designed (for example, equipment failure). Such special causes result in an "unstable" process. Another type of variation is *common-cause variation*, which arises from the way a process is designed. Such a process is said to be "stable" or in statistical "control"—that is, performing within a predictable range. That range, however, may not be what the organization desires. To reduce common-cause variation, design changes are necessary for the process being examined. The control chart in Figure 2-4, page 60, illustrates an unstable process, the same process brought under control, and that process's performance once design changes are made.

Statistical assessment also can show causal links. For example, a Pareto chart illustrates the frequency of events to illustrate possible causes of current performance (see Figure 2-5, page 61). A Pareto chart often shows that relatively few causes result in the majority of undesirable outcomes. For another example, a scatter diagram can be used to illustrate the relationship between two variables (see Figure 2-6, page 62). Statistical assessment can also show patterns and trends in performance and whether they are statistically significant. A run chart is one tool used to illustrate such patterns and trends (see Figure 2-7, page 63).

Once raw patient input has been turned into useful information about performance, that information can be put to use

Figure 2-4. Control Chart: Patient Waiting Time for Admission

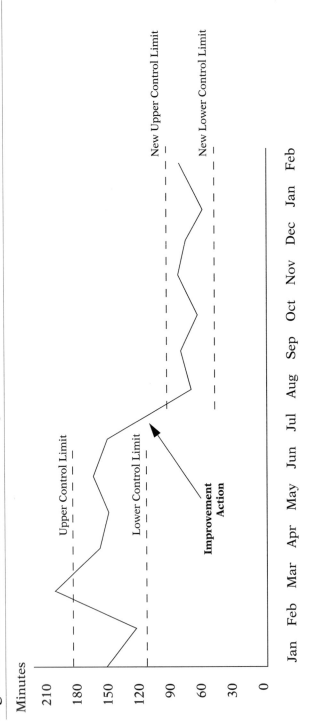

Figure 2-4. *This hypothetical control chart illustrates a process that is, at first, out of statistical control and that is performing outside the organization's targets. After bringing the process under control, improvement actions are possible. These actions shift the rate of performance, creating new upper and lower control limits.*

Figure 2-5. Pareto Chart: Patient Waiting Time for Admission

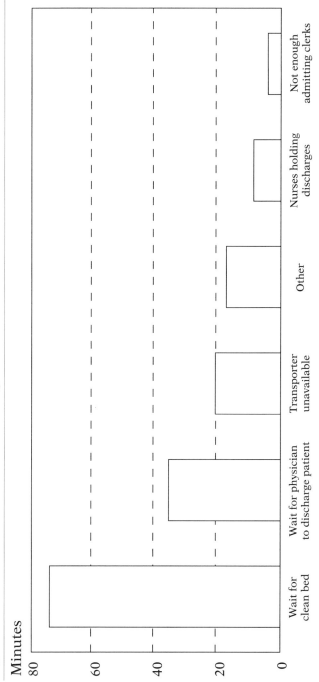

Figure 2-5. *A Pareto chart shows the frequency of events being studied in descending order. Often a Pareto chart is used to illustrate that a few causes are responsible for the majority of outcomes.*

Figure 2-6. Scatter Diagram: Patient Waiting Time Versus "Hospital occupancy"

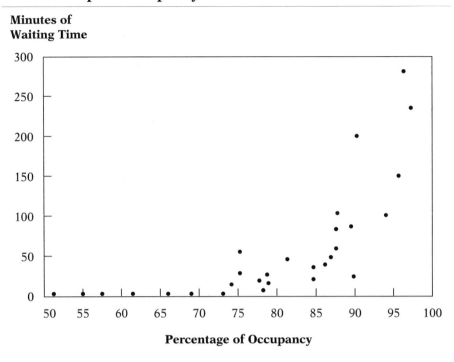

Figure 2-6. *A scatter diagram compares two variables—in this case, patient waiting time and hospital occupancy—to determine the relationship. Here, the clustering of points shows that census affects waiting time.*

improving performance. If the assessment addresses patient input that is being collected continuously, the assessment might suggest that a process is performing satisfactorily and needs no special attention, or it might show that a more intensive measurement, assessment, and improvement effort is warranted. Assessment of patient input as part of such an intensive effort should result in the translation of that patient input into improvement actions.

Improve

Improvement may mean designing a new process, or it may mean redesigning an existing process. Both improvement efforts

Figure 2-7. Run Chart: Average Length of Stay

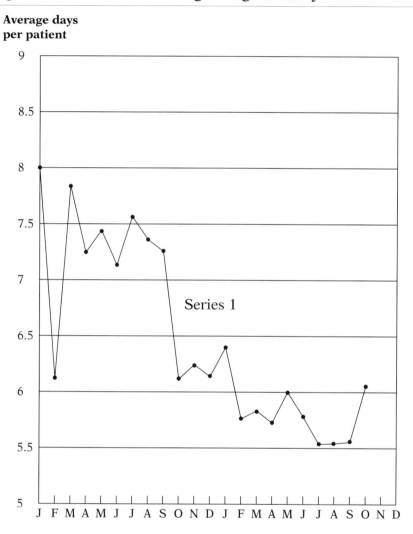

Average days per patient

Series 1

J F M A M J J A S O N D J F M A M J J A S O N D

Figure 2-7. *This figure shows how a run chart is used to display levels of performance over time—in this case, the average length of stay per patient over two years.*

can be fueled by patient input. For example, input from AIDS patients (along with other considerations, such as community needs and organizational mission) may influence an organization to create a community outreach program for people with AIDS—that is, design a new process. Waiting time involved in same-day surgery admission might encourage a hospital to examine its current admission process and make modifications to reduce waiting time—that is, redesign the existing process.

Whether using patient input to design a new process or redesign an existing process, the goal is to translate patient input into specific characteristics that can be addressed by the design or redesign. (Such characteristics are sometimes called "key quality characteristics," "design specifications," or "process, service, or product requirements.") Of course, not all characteristics of a process will be based on patient input (patient input would not, for example, determine postsurgical antibiotic administration); however, patient input can and should influence a range of important characteristics in many health care processes.

In preparing to design a new process or redesign an existing process, Thomas P. Nolan, PhD, a consultant with Associates in Process Improvement, suggests that teams consider the following three questions:

- What is the aim or purpose of the design or redesign effort? The answer to this question focuses attention on the goals of the initiative and creates a common purpose.

- How will we know the effort is successful? The answer to this question yields the measures of performance for the process.

Some patient needs require reanalysis of current practice patterns. "For example, many patients crave information at times when no one authorized to give it is available. Delegating authority to provide more information on the spot is called for even though this will challenge long traditions of tight heirarchical control over who can provide certain information.. Other serious problems such as long waiting times for pain medication, are amenable to technological solutions: providing self-administered analgesics is an easier solution. . ."

—excerpted from article by
Thomas W. Moloney and Barbara Paul
Health Affairs, Winter 1991, p 276

- For a redesign effort, what are the changes we can make and test that will lead to improvement? For a new process, how should the process be designed, what are the key characteristics, and how will we test the new process? The answers to these questions provide a menu of potential actions that should result in performance improvement. These improvement ideas are generated by the individuals who are closest to the work and understand, through their experience, the operations of the key work processes.

To ensure that patient input is part of the improvement effort, consider how information about patient needs, wants, perceptions, and so on can be incorporated into the answers to each of the three questions listed above.

Purpose of the improvement effort

A central purpose of almost any improvement effort in a health care organization is to better serve patients. Therefore, when articulating the aim or purpose of the improvement effort, it is important to include the effects on patient, and view those effects from the patient's perspective.

Knowing when redesign or design is successful

The success of an improvement effort must, at least in part, reflect how it has improved patient care or service. Therefore, when identifying the indicators with which the new or redesigned process will be measured, some should require patient input. These indicators can be derived from the patient input that was collected and assessed at this point in the improvement cycle.

Taking Action

To ensure that patient input is part of the actual improvement initiative, the team should translate patient input into specific characteristics for the new design or design changes. These characteristics can be derived from needs assessments and other patient input.

A well-known method to make improvements that addresses the three questions above is the Plan-Do-Study-Act (PDSA) cycle. This cycle, developed by Walter Shewhart and widely taught by W. Edwards Deming, is illustrated in Figure 2-8, page 67.

The *plan* stage in the cycle involves creating an operational plan for testing the chosen improvement action. Small-scale testing is necessary to determine whether an improvement action is viable, whether it will have the desired result, and whether any refinements are necessary before putting the action into full operation. Planning involves determining who will be involved in the test, what they need to know to participate in the test, the testing timetables, how the test will be implemented, why the idea is being tested, what the success factors are, and how the process and outcomes of the test will be measured and assessed.

The *do* stage involves implementing the pilot test and collecting actual performance data. *Study* (sometimes called *check*) means analyzing the data collected during the pilot test. This analysis seeks to learn whether the improvement action was entirely successful, partially successful, or unsuccessful in achieving the desired outcome(s). To determine the degree of success, compare actual test performance to desired performance targets and to baseline results achieved using the usual process. If the tested improvement action was unsuccessful, it is necessary to return to the plan stage.

The *act* stage involves implementing the changes if the tests are successful. The effectiveness of the new or redesigned process continues to be measured and assessed.

Tools for Making Improvements

Because improvements are a natural outgrowth of measurement and assessment, the tools used in those activities may also

Figure 2-8. PDSA Cycle

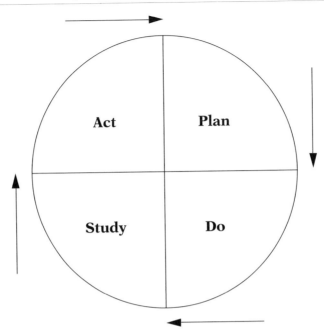

Figure 2-8. *This cycle—also called the Shewhart Cycle—is useful in planning, testing, assessing, and implementing an action to improve a process.*

SOURCE: Shewhart WA: Economic Control of Quality Manufactured Product. *New York: Van Nostrand, 1931.*

play a role in improvement. For example,

- *brainstorming* can be used to create ideas for improvement actions;
- *selection grids* can help a group decide among possible improvement actions (see Figure 2-9, page 68);
- *flowcharts* can help a group design a new process or redesign an existing one (see Figure 2-10, pages 69 and 70);
- *Pareto charts* can show the effect of improvement actions on root causes; and
- *run charts* and *control charts* can measure the effect of a process change.

Figure 2-9. Selection Grid: Setting Improvement Priorities

Decision Factor / Process	High-volume	High-risk	Problem-prone	Importance to organization mission	Importance to patients	Effect on costs	TOTAL
Admission/Discharge							
Emergency Dept Patient Flow							
Total Hip Replacement							
C-Section							
AIDS Education							
Bacterial Pneumonia Care							
. . .							

KEY TO SCORING:
X = strong effect   X = 3
O = some effect   O = 2
— = weak effect   — = 1
= no effect   = 0

Figure 2-9. *This figure shows a selection grid—a matrix used to weigh decision factors and help a group reach consensus. This example shows how a selection grid could be used to help a health care organization set priorities for its improvement efforts. Each person involved in making the decision assigns scores indicating how heavily each decision factor applies to each process the organization is considering targeting for improvement. Once the scores are totaled, they should indicate the priorities for improvement.*

SOURCE: Based on Kano SN, et al: Attractive Quality and Must-Be Quality. Methuen, MA: GOAL-QPC. 1984

Figure 2-10. Before-and-After Flowcharts: Room Cleaning

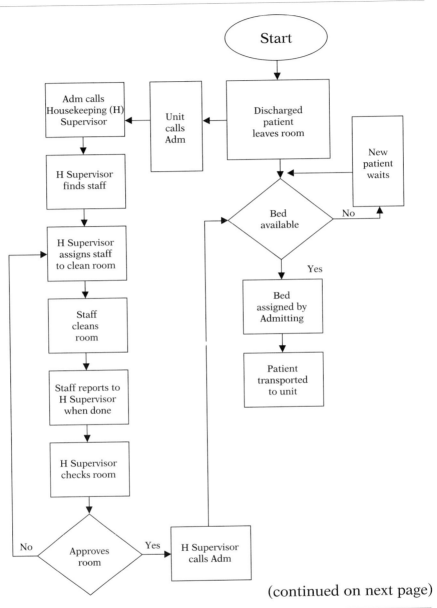

(continued on next page)

Figure 2-10. *A flowchart is an excellent way to learn about an existing process, to redesign an existing process, and to design a new process. This figure shows the process for room cleaning after a patient is discharged and before a new patient is transported to his or her room. The figure on this page is the existing process; the figure on page 70 is the redesigned process.*

Figure 2-10. Before-and-After Flowcharts: Room Cleaning (*continued*)

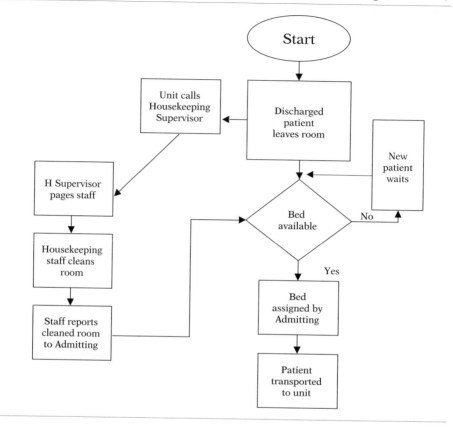

Using Patient Input to Improve Performance

There are several ways to approach the task of translating patient input into characteristics for a new design or the redesign of an existing process. Often, health care organizations consult experts at this stage. The following steps, which are based in part on the techniques used in Quality Function Deployment, illustrate one possible method. This method involves the following activities:

- Organize patient requirements;
- Rank requirements according to importance;

- Translate patient input into design characteristics; and

- Develop indicators or measures.

Organize patient requirements

Because patients will not deliver a categorized list of needs for the design of a given process, staff need to spend time sorting and organizing patient input into "groups of similar concerns." Content analysis is a good tool for this task.

The dimensions of performance discussed on page 38–39, and defined in Table 2-2, may be helpful in organizing patient input into logical groups. To review, those dimensions are efficacy, appropriateness, availability, effectiveness, timeliness, safety, efficiency, continuity, and respect and caring. Most patient needs will fall under one or more of these dimensions. Staff members can refine these categories by adding subcategories under each dimension.

Rank requirements according to importance

The specific information from patient input can be ranked according to the importance placed on it by the patient (for example, from 1 to 10). A Pareto chart (see Figure 2-5), which can display the information in descending order by importance, is a useful tool for displaying these data.

Translate patient input into process specifications

Once appropriate staff members have assessed data—patient input as well as other data about how a process is performing—they can translate that information into characteristics of the new process or of the redesigned process. Patient needs, expectations, and other input should be built into the actual steps used to carry out a process. A flowchart is an excellent tool for illustrating the steps in a process and the relationship of those steps (see Figure 2-10).

For example, a team assigned to expand an organization's current pediatric services to include pediatric rehabilitation might discover that parents worry about transporting their children back and forth to clinic visits, physical therapy, and so forth. Translated into a specification, this need might be expressed as "access to rehabilitation services."

During redesign efforts, staff reexamine current specifications in light of patient research. For example, a team assessing the process for ordering lab tests might discover that many patients feel confused by the number of lab tests ordered and that they would like to know the purpose of tests. As a result of this research, the team might expand the existing process specifications to include "patient education provided."

The matrix provided in Figure 2-11, page 73, can be used to translate patient input into design characteristics.

Develop indicators and measure performance of the new process

Measures of performance must be developed so the team can determine how the new or changed process is performing. Patient needs and expectations should be used to create these measures. (Developing indicators to measure performance is discussed in the "measure" section of this chapter.) In most cases, the patient needs and expectations that were translated into characteristics of the

66 *The emerging science of patient care could spawn a generation of patient-interactive technologies, including educational material on the risks and rewards of treatment options and on self-management of chronic disease, as well as survey information on patients' assessments of competing medical groups, hospitals, and medical care plans. Patient-administered and monitored treatments should also become commonplace. . . .* 99

—excerpted from Karl Albrecht: *The Only Thing That Matters.* NYC: *Harper Business,* 1992

Figure 2-11. Matrix for Translating Patient Input into Process Characteristics

Service/Process: Mammograms

Dimension	Patient Input Verbatim	Rank	Process/Service Specification	Indicator	Question(s) on Satisfaction Survey
Example: Safety	*I don't want to be exposed to unnecessary radiation*	3	*Lead aprons are used for all mammograms.*	*Was a lead apron used? Yes/No*	*Did you feel that you were protected from unnecessary radiation?*
Example: Timeliness	*I don't want to wait.*	6	*Patient is seen within x minutes of appointment time.*	*Did the patient wait more than x minutes past their appointment time?*	*Did you feel that you had to wait too long?*
Appropriateness					
Availability					
Effectiveness					
Efficacy					
Efficiency					
Example: Continuity	*I want to know the results as soon as possible.*	2	*Mammogram to physician in 48 hours.* *Physician to call patient in 72 hours.*	*Did physician get report within 48 hours?* *Did physician call patient within 72 hours?*	*Did you receive a call from the physician in an acceptable time frame?*
Example: Respect and Caring	*I want to know what is happening to me and why I'm having this procedure.*	5	*Physician explains why this test is being ordered.* *Technician explains what is happening as mammogram is being performed.*	*Did the physician discuss the purpose of the mammogram with the patient?* *Did the technician explain the procedure to the patient?*	*Did you understand why you had this mammogram and what was going on during the test?*

Figure 2-11. *Staff can use this matrix when translating patient input into key characteristics to be designed into a process. From these specifications, indicators can be developed to measure whether the actions taken satisfied patients.*

process can be written as performance measures. Teams may not be able to measure all process characteristics. They may choose to measure only those specifications that were found to be most important to patients.

Once a new or redesigned process has been implemented, teams must measure its effect. This measurement often involves going back to patients and collecting feedback to see if the process is meeting their needs and expectations. The most common way to test patient satisfaction is through a written or telephone survey. To develop an instrument to measure satisfaction, staff can return to the specifications and indicators they developed based on patient needs and expectations (see Figure 2-11). Survey questions can then be developed for each indicator staff chose to measure.

If the results of the satisfaction survey indicate that the improvement was not effective in meeting patient needs and expectations, staff members will need to rethink the situation and develop and test a new plan of action. Only when the organization is satisfied with the results of the trial, should a new or redesigned process be fully implemented. Then, measurement and periodic assessment should continue to examine the process's long-term effect.

Next Step

This discussion of performance improvement, with special attention to patient input, should provide a theoretical framework that can help organizations use patient input to improve organizational performance. The specific examples in Chapter 3 should help health care professionals see how the cycle for improving performance can be tailored to a particular organization's needs. Chapter 3 also provides four examples of how organizations carry out patient-focused and customer-focused improvement activities.

References

1. Quinn D: Principles of data collection applied to customer knowledge. *J Healthc Qual* 14(6): 24–36, Nov/Dec 1992.

2. Day RG: *Quality Function Deployment: Linking a Company With Its Customers*. Milwaukee, WI: ASQC Press, 1993, p 40.

3. Joint Commission on Accreditation of Healthcare Organizations: *The Measurement Mandate: On the Road to Performance Improvement in Health Care*. Oakbrook Terrace, IL, 1993, p 255.

Chapter 3

Using Patient Input to Improve Performance—

Four Examples

The following four case studies demonstrate how health care organizations have put the concepts expressed in the previous chapters into practice. Each example addresses a different facet of care; each illustrates a distinct method for collecting the input from patients and putting that information to use in improving care. Despite these differences, these four examples have much in common. All place a premium on the view of patients and other customers; all lay out a method for measurement, assessment, and improvement; and all show a quest for continuous improvement.

Example 1: Patient Information About Breast Cancer

This example shows how one organization gathered and examined patient input about breast cancer information, assessed current resources and processes, and designed a new process to fulfill this crucial patient need.

The University of Wisconsin Hospitals (UWH) in Madison wanted to improve its provision of care to women with breast cancer.[1,2] According to David Gustafson, professor in industrial engineering and preventive medicine at the university, UWH decided to focus on the informational needs of breast cancer patients because of "evidence suggesting that information (for example, what the experience will be like and how to cope with it) and support lead to more accurate expectations, improved health status, increased longevity among breast cancer patients, and improved health status among their primary supporters."[2]

In developing the breast cancer needs assessment study, Gustafson decided to use a combination of two methods. The critical incident technique was used to explore patients' needs and expectations. Then, from the data obtained, a written survey was developed. Responses to this survey allowed UWH staff to determine those needs that were most important to breast cancer patients.

First, Gustafson selected an expert panel consisting of two women with breast cancer, two adult daughters of women with breast cancer, two partners of women with breast cancer, one breast cancer surgeon, one nurse practitioner in the breast clinic, and two nurse researchers. The providers were asked to participate in the panel to provide advice about patient needs and, more importantly, to allow them to hear what patients had to say. (Since its original formation, the panel was expanded to include one radiation oncologist and one medical oncologist.)

Next, Gustafson conducted phone interviews with each panel member. Each interview lasted about 45 minutes. He asked panel members to describe each step in the disease process from her or his own perspective. In these interviews, Gustafson was looking for "critical incidents" or key episodes. For example, when asking the two women with breast cancer about their time of diagnosis, he asked them to think of the time the physician walked in the room and said, "I have bad news." "What was it like? What fears did you have? Frustrations? Barriers? Uncertainties? What thoughts ran through your head? What stands out in your mind?"

The critical incident technique asks patients to think about a specific event and describe the critical incidents that come to mind. The interviewer continues to prompt the respondent until the critical incidents become clear. For example, a patient might say, "I can remember the drains. Nobody told me what it would be like to be on drains. You cannot imagine how humiliating it is to walk outside and have these drains hanging out below your coat. I was so embarrassed that I couldn't go outside." When Gustafson received that sort of comment, he would not stop. He would ask the respondent why that was such a difficult thing for her, why it stands out in her mind so much. She might then say, "It was just such a dramatic signal that I was sick."

Gustafson said that interviewing different players in the disease process helps create what he refers to as "joint discovery." For example, when he asked the patient what it was like to learn she had cancer, she might say, "I remember sitting in the doctor's office and having her talk to me about the diagnosis. And, you know, I didn't hear a word she said." Then, when Gustafson interviewed the physician about the same step in the process, she said "I know they're not listening. I know they're not hearing what I have to say. It goes in one ear and out the other. They're not ready to hear me. They're too shocked." If different people involved in the process say essentially the same thing, staff can begin to detect patterns and trends.

After the telephone interviews were completed, Gustafson brought the panel members together. The information obtained from the interviews had been classified, organized, and displayed on flip charts around the room. Panel members were then asked if any needs were left off the charts, whether any information had been misinterpreted, and so forth. From this meeting, the panel came up with a list of potential needs.

From this list, three pilot surveys were created (one for women with breast cancer, one for daughters, and one for husbands). These surveys were then distributed to a breast cancer support group called the "Bosom Buddies." Gustafson asked the Bosom Buddies to fill out the survey for women with breast cancer and have their daughters and husbands fill out the other two surveys. He also asked them to note any wording that was inaccurate, any additional questions they felt should be on the survey, and so forth.

From this pilot test, staff revised the surveys. Examples of the types of issues the survey asked women with breast cancer to rate included: What should a good insurance policy cover? What can I do about switching insurance when I have preexisting conditions? When will it be safe to have sex? How can I deal with body image? How can I deal with children's reactions to finding that I had breast cancer? (See Appendix C, pages 127–151, for a sample of this survey.)

UWH wanted to include other hospitals besides their own in the study. Six other hospitals agreed to collect data from 30 women with breast cancer, 30 partners, and 30 adult daughters. To assess patient needs at different points in the disease process, the surveys were distributed to respondents at three times— diagnosis, three months later, and nine months later. Patients were not followed over time. Four hundred completed surveys were returned by the hospitals.

In analyzing the results from the breast cancer needs survey, staff learned that in terms of the importance of information provided to them, "prospect of recovery" was rated the highest by all groups. Information about sexuality was rated as the least important.

When these findings were presented to staff in the participating hospitals, they said, "We used to meet those needs before DRGs [diagnosis related groups]. We're getting pressured and have to do all these technical medical things. We don't have time to deal with those kind of issues." Gustafson and his staff realized that the human resources were not there to meet these patient needs. They also realized that a lot of the problems these patients had arose at any time of day or night. Thus, they needed a process that provided information to patients when they needed it.

UWH now offers each woman diagnosed with breast cancer a computer to take home for three months. The computer includes an interactive program called CHESS, which includes several applications for patients to use that were developed based on feedback from the needs assessment survey. A database provides answers to 200 commonly asked questions by breast cancer patients; an instant library includes up-to-date articles and pamphlets on breast cancer; a decision aid helps patients think through difficult decisions (such as, chemotherapy versus hormonal therapy); and a discussion group allows women to interact with other breast cancer patients through electronic mail. Because patients can take these computers home with them, they can access this information at any time, whether it is three o'clock in the afternoon or two o'clock in the morning.

UWH conducted two pilot studies for CHESS using five adult daughters and ten women with breast cancer. Changes were made

> 66 *The emerging science of patient care could spawn a generation of patient-interactive technologies, including educational material on the risks and rewards of treatment options and on self-management of chronic disease, as well as survey information on patients' assessments of competing medical groups, hospitals, and medical care plans. Patient-administered and monitored treatments should also become commonplace. . . .* 99
>
> —from Thomas W. Moloney and Barbara Paul: Rebuilding public trust and confidence. In Gerteis M: *Through the Patient's Eyes.* San Francisco: Jossey-Bass Publishers, 1993, p 295.

based on the results of these pilot tests. Then staff beta-tested CHESS by offering it to women as they left the surgeon's office regardless of their age and education. During these tests, all users found that "CHESS created positive emotions (such as empathy and empowerment) and did not create negative emotions (such as fear and boredom)."

Encouraged by these tests, the Department of Surgery at UWH made CHESS a "mandated service" for all breast cancer surgery patients in January 1993. Staff also plan to study CHESS on a wider scale as soon as possible.

Example 2: Pain Management

This example shows how a hospital's efforts at patient-centered care led to significant redesign of the pain-management process. The hospital used patient input to make important modifications to existing practices. Continued collection of patient input demonstrates that the redesigned process has had good results.

Parkland Memorial Hospital in Dallas began its pain-management study as a result of the hospital's involvement in the Picker-Commonwealth Patient-Centered Care Program. According to Karen Cawley, senior vice president of surgical services, an initial Picker-Commonwealth survey revealed that 70% of Parkland's surgical patients reported experiencing pain while in the hospital. Eighty percent of those described their pain as moderate or severe, and 25% of those patients believed their pain could have been eliminated or better handled by more timely attention from staff.

Cawley and her staff decided to focus the initial redesign activity in the orthopedic unit and the burn acute care unit, which is a step-down unit from the intensive care area. Pain management at Parkland is handled in the following way: on these units (as on most units), a typical physician's order for pain medication may be "morphine sulphate, 5–15 mg IM, q3–4 hours prn pain." Based on his or her assessment of the patient, the nurse may then decide how much medication to administer and how frequently to administer it within these parameters.

Both Cawley and Ann Honaker, director of surgical acute care, suspected that the high percentage of patients who complained about pain was due in part to biases and attitudes on the part of nurses, which influenced their decisions to give pain medication. Their hypothesis was supported by studies in the literature indicating that physicians tend to underprescribe pain medication, and nurses tend to undermedicate patients in pain. "I think medicine is still quite paternalistic," Cawley said. "Many nurses and physicians believe that they are better judges or more appropriate judges of patients' pain, and need for pain medication, than the patients themselves."

Honaker said staff had several goals for the pain-management study. They wanted to collect information on the effectiveness of Parkland's current pain-management practices. They also wanted to evaluate how much the nurses knew about effective pain management and test their hypothesis that attitudes and biases regarding pain management influenced nursing practice. Finally, they wanted to look at patient charts to see how much pain-management medication nurses were giving to patients.

They approached each objective separately. A survey developed by three experts in pain management specifically tested nurse attitudes and biases in this area. All the nurses in the two pilot units were asked to complete the survey. A separate interview tool, developed by a pain research group at the University of Wisconsin, was used to interview a sample of patients on both units about their perceptions of their pain. Also, a chart audit tool was developed, and staff evaluated charts in the burn acute care unit to see how much medication had been ordered and how much medication was actually given.

The results of the nurses' survey and the chart audit supported Honaker and Cawley's hypothesis—many nurses demonstrated attitudes and biases that caused them to be less sensitive to patients' need for pain medication. The chart audit indicated that many of the surveyed patients who reported their pain as being severe were not given the full range of medication that physicians prescribed.

As the next phase of the study, nurses on the two units were required to attend a full-day education program on pain management and/or view videotapes on the subject. Presenting the results of the study to the nurses also affected their attitudes. Honaker said it was helpful to "go to the nurses and say, 'Mr X said his pain was really quite bad but you chose to give him the least amount of pain medication possible.' It was really an eye opener to them."

On the burn unit, the manager also chose to institute pain-management protocols. These protocols require nurses to regularly ask patients about their pain. Nurses then indicate on the protocol the amount of medication to give patients depending on the patients' level of pain.

After the nurses completed the education program, they were resurveyed to see if any of their attitudes and biases about pain management had changed. A second round of interviews was conducted with patients, and chart audits were again completed.

Although the second chart audit did not demonstrate that patients were receiving more medication, patients indicated during interviews that they perceived their pain to be less. Patients reported that nurses were inquiring more frequently and more regularly about their pain, as the protocol required. Although uncertain what the cause of this finding may be, Honaker suspects it may be related to the halo effect: "Nurses are asking patients about their pain and so they are more comfortable."

Realizing it is difficult to change attitudes quickly, Cawley and Honaker believe more improvement still needs to be made in the area of pain management. Future plans call for individual nursing units to initiate additional educational programs and develop unit protocols relating to the assessment of pain and the administration of pain medication. Also, the department of surgical services is developing a plan to form a multidisciplinary pain-management team, coordinated by a nurse clinical specialist and composed of nurses, physicians, and pharmacists, to design and implement a departmental pain-management program.

Example 3. Reengineering for Patient-Centered Care

—Developed and written by Francis A. Fullam, Director of Organizational Transformation, University of Chicago Hospitals, Chicago.

This example shows an effort to use patient input to improve care that spans not only a large hospital, but an alliance of academic medical centers. The method used is broad enough to apply across a range of hospital units and departments—and to incorporate information from other hospitals. This example describes the overall method for using patient input, with some specific illustrations from certain patient care units.

Most U.S. hospitals, whether they want to or not, are in the process of reengineering themselves because of the rapidly changing health care environment. At the University of Chicago Hospitals, a 637-bed academic medical center in Chicago, we were concerned about cost and efficiency issues facing all hospitals. But we also believe that an increase in medical specialization and emphasis on technology have caused the patient to slip from the focus of concern in health care. We wanted to balance both issues at the same time. We call our effort to simultaneously change our institutional culture and operating efficiency "The Transformation." The name embodies our need to lower our costs and become more patient centered. We are very clear about this in the Hospital's statement of purpose: "On a foundation of mutual respect, we will work together to build the University of Chicago Hospitals into one of the finest organizations in the country—as measured by the satisfaction of each patient, the efficiency of the organization and the level of pride among everyone who works here."

To demonstrate how serious we are about patient-centered care, we have tied part of employee compensation to patient satisfaction scores. Certain units and departments of the hospital have specific targets, and there are substantial bonuses if they meet those targets. However, if the units or departments do not meet the targets, managers do not get the bonus.

We have found the work of the Picker Institute to be extremely helpful. The program provides an invaluable framework for thinking about patients' concerns. Their seven dimensions of patient-centered care gave us a language that everyone in health care services can share. These dimensions are:

- Respect for patients' values;

- Transition and continuity of care;

- Information and education;

- Involvement of family and friends;

- Physical comfort;

66One consulting group's experimental model for patient-focused care has decentralized such ancillary patient care services as admissions, radiology, pharmacy, and routine laboratory work to the unit level and has cross-trained nurses in phlebotomy, physical therapy, and respiratory therapy. The model unit has also redesigned physical space to bring supplies and services closer to the patient and has coordinated all activities through patient care 'partnerships' headed by nurses.**99**

—from Margaret Gerteis: Coordinating care and integrating services. In Gerteis M: *Through the Patient's Eyes*. San Francisco: Jossey-Bass Publishers, 1993, p 65.

- Emotional support; and
- Coordination of care.

We are forming multidisciplinary teams on different units across the hospitals to implement patient-centered care. Essentially the units follow three steps:

- Develop guidelines for the way the caregivers want to deliver care;
- Measure or survey whether patients feel we are providing good care; and
- Develop a system for providing feedback to caregivers about their performance.

Each of these steps is described in further detail in the following paragraphs.

Developing Guidelines

Five-North is a 48-bed general medicine unit selected to pilot-test new approaches to patient-centered care. A multidisciplinary team, with representatives from all groups providing care and service on the unit, worked together to develop practice guidelines. The guidelines apply to all those providing care and service and set forth clear expectations for the manner in which care is delivered. The following are examples of some of the guidelines established on 5 North:

- Patients should be addressed by the names they want to be called;
- Always knock on the door or announce yourself before entering a patient room; and
- Health care professionals should explain the purpose, action, and timing of medications and treatments of patients.

The multidisciplinary teams used the dimensions of patient-centered care in developing their guidelines. One tool that was used to stimulate discussion about guidelines is the "Patient-Centered Care Guidelines Worksheet" (Figure 3-1, page 89). The tool is simply a matrix; the dimensions are listed vertically and the caregivers are listed horizontally. A facilitator worked with each team to fill out the matrix.

The teams also use many tools and techniques of total quality management (TQM), including cause-and-effect diagrams, multivoting, and so forth. However, we do not call ourselves a TQM hospital. Since we have been striving to provide quality care since our founding, we did not feel it was necessary to formally call ourselves a "quality" hospital. Instead, we work TQM tools and techniques into reengineering activities. When teams encounter a problem, the facilitator shows members the tools. However, we do not burden people with the jargon of the technique.

For example, on 5 North, we found some patient-provider communication problems. We found that care providers addressed patients by the name they wanted to be called only about 70% of the time. About 30% of the time, patients said that they were called, for example, Mary instead of Mrs Smith. The survey results helped change the perception of staff. They no longer assume they know what patients want to be called. Now, we meet patient expectations about 90% the time.

Measuring Patient Opinion

The University of Chicago Hospitals is a member of the University Hospital Consortium (UHC), an alliance of 65 academic medical centers, which is based in Oak Brook, Illinois. In 1991, we found that many members of the consortium were dissatisfied with our current patient satisfaction surveys. A group of us decided to design a new survey that we could all use and that would be the basis for a comparative database on patient satisfaction.

We adapted the Picker Institute survey, which asks patients

Figure 3-1. Patient-Centered Care Guidelines Worksheet

Dimension of patient-centered care	Nurse	Faculty	Housestaff	Allied Health Professionals	House-keepers	Social Workers
Respect for patient's values, preferences, and expressed needs						
Coordination of care						
Information and education						
Physical comfort						
Emotional support and alleviation of fear and anxiety						
Involvement of friends and family						
Continuity and transition of care						

Figure 3-1. *This matrix helps specific disciplines develop patient-centered guidelines pertaining to specific dimensions of care.*

to report on (rather than rate) aspects of their care. The main change we made was to shift the instrument from a telephone survey to a mail survey to obtain more responses for less money. Each hospital was also able to add organization-specific questions to their own survey. (See Figure 3-2, pages 91 and 92, for some sample questions from the survey.)

In 1992, we fielded our first survey and are currently in our third cycle. We have surveyed over 60,000 patients at 50 hospitals around the country. The University of Chicago Hospitals can now compare itself to these other hospitals in general and at the service level as well. We are able to say, "Here's what cancer patients at the University of Chicago think about their care. And here is what cancer patients think about their care at the University of X," and so on. This helps us identify opportunities for improvement. The ability to make service-level comparisons really engages the attention of our physicians.

This UHC database has allowed us to do some comparative benchmarking. All the hospitals in the consortium are willing to share information about best practices. For example, when we found out we did not do as well as we wanted on questions related to pain management, we looked into the hospital that had the best scores on pain management and found out that the hospital had a tremendous number of patient-controlled analgesia (PCA) pumps. We found we lagged behind this hospital in the ratio of PCA pumps to patients. As a result, our department of anesthesiology greatly increased the number of pumps and their availability. We quickly saw our pain scores go from below average to the same ranges as other hospitals.

Sharing Feedback

The first step in getting people to use patient feedback is to convince them that there is a problem. The best way to provide feedback depends on the group. For example, we provide nurses with satisfaction data by geographic unit. Physicians tend to want

Figure 3-2. Sample Questions from the University Hospital Consortium's Patient Survey

1. How often were doctors available to answer your questions and concerns when you needed them?

I had no questions or concerns	1
Always	2
Usually	3
Sometimes	4
Rarely	5
Never	6
Not sure	7

2. Was there ever a time when you felt that your:

   A. Doctors weren't talking to each other **enough about your case?**

Yes, definitely	1
Yes, somewhat	2
No	3
Not sure	4

   B. Doctors weren't talking with your nurses enough about your case?

Yes, definitely	1
Yes, somewhat	2
No	3
Not sure	4

3. Did you doctors discuss your anxieties or fears about your condition with you?

Yes, completely	1
Yes, somewhat	2
No	3
Not sure	4

4. When you had an important question to ask a nurse, how often did you get answers you could understand?

I had no important questions	1
Always	2
Usually	3
Sometimes	4
Rarely	5
Never	6
Not sure	7

(continued on next page)

Figure 3-2. Continued

5. When you needed help going to the bathroom, how often did you get it in time?

Never needed help	1
Always got it	2
Usually got it	3
Sometimes got it	4
Rarely got it	5
Never got it	6

6. Did the surgeon explain the risks and benefits of the surgery in a way you could understand?

Yes, completely	1
Yes, somewhat	2
No	3
Not sure	4

7. Did the hospital staff do everything they could to eliminate your pain, or do you think they could have done more?

Did everything they could	1
Could have done a little more	2
Could have done a lot more	3
Not sure	4

8. Did someone explain the purpose of each medicine you were told to take when you went home in a way that you could understand?

Yes, completely	1
Yes, somewhat	2
No	3
Not sure	4

9. If you needed additional care after leaving the hospital, did the hospital staff do all they could to help arrange for this care?

Yes, completely	1
Yes, somewhat	2
No	3
Not sure	4

10. Did you have enough say about your medical treatment in the hospital?

Yes, definitely	1
Yes, probably	2
No	3
Not sure	4

more statistical comparative information according to services. With the UHC survey, we are able to provide them with information that is service specific. We have found that you really cannot engage their attention until you get down to that level of detail. Physicians do not want to know about comparisons of medicine to surgery. They want to know how their patients do compared to similar patients in similar institutions.

Conclusion

Staff often argue that they need "more staff or more money" to make patients happy. The results of the UHC survey have shown that this simply is not true. With the UHC comparative database, we were able to compare the efficiency of each hospital, through some statistical measures of efficiency, with patient satisfaction ratings. We found that hospitals designed to operate more efficiently tend to have higher patient satisfaction scores. If you have a process in place that takes care of patients efficiently (for example, they are not forced to wait long periods of time), these patients tend to be more satisfied.

Example 4: Quality Function Deployment: Listening to the Voice of the Customer

—Developed and written by Eric W. Kratochwill, Senior Staff Associate, and Deborah M. Ehrlich, PhD, Manager of Market Research, University of Michigan Medical Center, Ann Arbor, Michigan.

Like the previous example, this one shows an organization-wide approach to improvement. This approach, Quality Function Deployment (QFD), addresses not just input from patients, but input from other "customer" groups, including referring physicians, patients, payers, students, and employees, and medical staff. This approach emphasizes, among other things, the complex customer-supplier relationships that exist within an organization and between the organization and external groups.

Table 3-1. UMMC Patient Quality Indicators

Patients applaud the Medical Center when:

- Access and service are timely and convenient;

- Service and care are coordinated and efficient;

- Facilities are comfortable, clean, and attractive;

- They have the knowledge necessary to be comfortable in their environment and partners in their care;

- They are treated with respect;

- The expected clinical result is obtained; and

- The UMMC staff members are caring and compassionate.

The example that follows explains the steps in QFD, as well as how this approach came to be adopted at this organization. Each step in QFD can be applied to patients, but can be most productively employed by using input from all relevant customer groups, including patients. Therefore, this examples highlights input from patients and other customers.

The University of Michigan Medical Center (UMMC) developed institutional quality indicators in 1990. These indicators allow the organization to measure the degree and frequency of conformity to customer requirements. The indicators serve as the foundation for UMMC's Total Quality Process (TQP). Through the tracking and analysis of these indicators, we are able to respond to specific customer requirements throughout the organization.

We developed indicators for each of our five customer groups: referring physicians, patients, payers, students and employees, and medical staff. Through focus groups with each customer type, we established clear, measurable indicators to track our success. The quality indicators for our patients are offered in Table 3-1 (above).

In our customer satisfaction surveys, we track our progress quantitatively for each indicator. The patient satisfaction survey process follows the Plan-Do-Check-Act (PDCA) process. Surveys are conducted once every two years so that departments have sufficient time to make changes and assess results. The survey process acts as a continual pretest and posttest measurement technique. The intention is to identify weak areas, make changes, and then see if the changes have been effective.

An example of this process comes from a recent survey that identified patients who did not perceive themselves as "partners in their care." In response, a quality improvement team focused on developing strategies for clinicians to include patients in their care. The team conducted focus groups to identify how patients define their role as partners in care. Based on this information, surveys were developed and sent to patients and the UMMC medical staff to measure satisfaction with, and expectations of, patients being partners in their care. The results will allow the team to identify gaps between

66*At Mayo . . . patients know what to expect during the course of their stay. Within an hour after their initial examination, they will know exactly what tests have been scheduled; exactly when and where they will take place; exactly how long they will take; and exactly what they will entail. . . One patient described, with gratitude, how his nurse 'took me under her wing [and] told me what to expect by the hour the next day.' Patients in New York University Hospital's Cooperative Care Unit are given daily schedules of their 'appointments' with doctors, nurses, and clinics, even though the schedules have to be revised and updated frequently.*99

—from Margaret Gerteis: Coordinating care and integrating services. In Gerteis M: *Through the Patient's Eyes*. San Francisco: Jossey-Bass Publishers, 1993, p 59.

patient and physician expectations. Finally, the team will develop a training program to educate the medical staff on how to enhance patient participation in their care.

Each department throughout the UMMC—clinical and non-clinical—is charged with developing two departmental quality indicators based on the institution's quality indicators. The coordinated tracking and improvement of the quality indicators help align the quality improvement efforts of all the departments and divisions throughout the institution.

The Quality Function Deployment Process at UMMC

In 1990, recognizing the challenge of meeting the requirements of all five customer groups, the UMMC decided to apply an advanced total quality technique called Quality Function Deployment. QFD was selected because it has been successful in various manufacturing industries. Numerous articles have documented the success of QFD in diverse industries (Akao, 1990[3]; Hauser and Clausing, 1988[4]; King, 1989[5]). The UMMC hoped the impressive results could be repeated in a service industry such as health care.

QFD was first used in the medical procedures unit (MPU), a multidisciplinary unit that combined adult and pediatric gastroenterology, pulmonary, and cardiac diagnostic and procedural services. The MPU was selected because it represented an opportunity to apply QFD in a unit that was consolidating previously separate services and customer groups into a single service. We hoped QFD would offer a new means to align resources to meet valid customer requirements. The ultimate goal was to stimulate service volume through enhanced patient and referring physician satisfaction.

The QFD process begins by identifying the key customer groups of the product or service. Focus group research among key customer groups is then conducted to obtain the "voice of the customer." The focus group transcripts are analyzed in detail, and the information is prioritized through a mathematical matrix. This complex matrix enables the organization to determine the most important customer requirments and the service attributes that will best meet those requirements. Customer requirements are then integrated into the design at the earliest stages of the process.

At first glance, QFD sounds similar to a typical marketing and planning process. However, QFD involves pooling the expertise of *all* departments that play a role in the success of the unit to align resources to meet customer requirements. The multidisciplinary group analyzes the verbatim comments of each customer group, prioritizes various requirements, determines the organization's strengths and weaknesses in these areas, compares these findings with competitors, and aligns the organization's resources to best meet the diverse customer expectations.

QFD is a complex process that requires extensive staff time and team member training. In addition, the team needs to be led by an experienced QFD facilitator or expert. Frequently, organizations dedicate internal consultants to serve as QFD professionals. Any organization undertaking QFD should realize that this is hard work, and it requires intense dedication of all team members.

The UMMC's experience with QFD has been challenging. Through internal training and help from an external consultant, the UMMC developed an eight-step QFD approach:

- Step 1: Identify customer groups;
- Step 2: Conduct customer focus groups;
- Step 3: Analyze the voice of the customer;
- Step 4: Verify customer priorities;
- Step 5: Determine priorities of customer requirements;
- Step 6: Analyze the organization's strengths and weaknesses;

- Step 7: Compare these findings to your competitors; and
- Step 8: Align resources to meet customer expectations.

The following paragraphs describe these steps as they have been carried out to date at the UMMC.

Step 1. Identify customer groups

The UMMC QFD team includes representatives from planning, marketing, administration, and finance and the clinical professionals involved in the MPU. The team identified four customer groups: MPU nurses, MPU staff physicians, referring physicians, and patients (see Figure 3-3, page 99). These groups represent external and internal customers of the MPU.

Step 2. Conduct customer focus groups

To obtain the "voice of the customer"—what the customer truly wants from the service—the team conducted focus groups for each specific customer group.

Step 3. Analyze the voice of the customer

To distill the "voice of the customer," the team critically analyzed the focus group transcripts line by line. Through this analysis, the multidisciplinary team identified what the customers said and the probable intent of what they said. Then the team distilled the essence of the customer requirement—they demanded quality. Examples of how the team distilled the demanded quality from referring physician and patient focus group comments are offered in Table 3-2, page 100.

The team used the "Voice of the Customer table" to critically analyze customer comments through a structured process. The team used this structured table to dissect each comment into basic customer requirements that are specific, positively stated, and actionable by the organization. As shown in Table 3-2, the original customer comments were interpreted into requirements

Figure 3-3. Medical Procedures Unit (MPU)Customer Groups

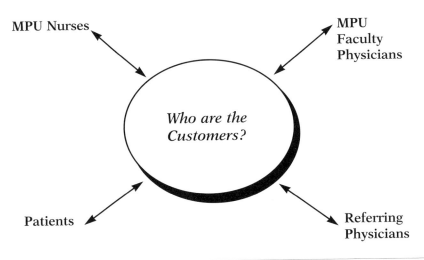

MPU Nurses

MPU
Faculty
Physicians

*Who are the
Customers?*

Patients

Referring
Physicians

Figure 3-3. *This figure illustrates the key customer groups identified by the medical procedures unit in its Quality Function Deployment initiative. The initiative continues by assessing the expectations these customers have for the unit.*

that the organization could concentrate on (that is, treat referring physicians respectfully or answer patient questions clearly).

An example from the auto industry may provide insight into the power of using this approach. An automobile company may hear, "I hate having to grope through my purse trying to find a key to get into my car . . . especially at night." A traditional approach to meeting customer demands might compel the company to design a larger key that would be easier to locate in a crowded purse. Or maybe the company would put a penlight on the key to enable the woman to see the lock easily at night. Both approaches appear to satisfy the customer's needs. However, a QFD team using the Voice of the Customer table would distill the true demanded quality: *to get into the car easily.* Stating the customer requirement in this way would enable the company to explore innovative approaches to meet this need, such as a numeric key pad that allows access to a car without any key.

Table 3-2. Voice of the Customer Table

Referring Physicians

Customer Comment	Reworded Data	Demanded Quality
At a university hospital, from the attending physician down to the residents, down to the interns, they don't care about the referring physician. They don't look at my prior workup. They only take you seriously if you know the specialist.	I want to be treated with respect.	Treat me respectfully.
	Treat me as a valuable client, even if I don't personally know the UMMC physician.	Respond to my request for services seriously.
	Review my workup before you treat my patient.	Value my professional judgment consistently.

Patients

Customer Comment	Reworded Data	Demanded Quality
I called the MPU to find out about my prep instructions and was transferred to multiple clinics.	I want my questions answered clearly.	Answer my prep questions promptly.
		Answer my prep questions competently.
		Provide a single point of contact for information.

Table 3-2. *This table shows how the "Voice of the customer table" translates customer comments into key quality demands that can then be made part of a new or redesigned process.*

Step 4. Verify customer priorities

Following this in-depth analysis of the customer's voice, the team developed affinity diagrams to identify themes and areas of major concern to customer groups. Then, based on the affinity diagram information, we developed survey instruments for each customer group to verify customer-demanded qualities. The surveys measured both satisfaction with each identified demanded quality and the need for change. We used this information to prioritize the numerous customer requirements.

Step 5. Determine priorities of customer requirements

The team then integrated the data into the "house of quality" matrix. The house of quality provides a structured means by which to prioritize customer requirements and identify the impact individual changes will have on multiple requirements. Through the use of the matrix, the team can also determine what changes will most successfully address various customer requirements. The matrix analysis is done using *QFD Capture* software.

Figure 3-4, page 102, is an example of a house-of-quality matrix. The team addressed the issue of communication with referring physicians and determined the relationships between the demanded qualities and the technical requirements—the elements of the existing processes that meet the requirements. Each relationship has a corresponding weight. Once all relationships are agreed on by the team, the matrix enables the team to determine quantitatively which technical requirement will have the greatest impact on the customer's demanded qualities. Through the matrix, the team uses a *quantitative* technique to translate qualitative customer demands into actionable strategies for improvement.

Figure 3-4. House of Quality Matrix

WHATs vs HOWs

Strong Relationship:	✪ 9
Medium Relationship:	● 3
Weak Relationship:	✳ 1

	Communicability (methods, types, and numbers of communication)	Report completeness and clarity	Clinical information availability (communications)	Staff availability to communicate	Timing of communication	Referral source accessibility	Referring physician patient information availability	Physician courtesy
UMMC communication w/referring physicians is timely	✪		✪	✪	✪	●	✳	✳
Completeness of patient information	✳	✪	✪		✳		✪	
House officers treat me respectfully	●	✳		✳	✪		●	✪
Informed about UMMC physicians to whom one can refer	●					✳	✳	
Able to contact UMMC physician easily	●			✪				✪
Patient information communicated concisely		✪	●	✳	●		●	
UMMC physician team values my (ref MD) professional judgment	✳				●	✳	✪	✪

Figure 3-4. *This matrix identifies the strengths of the relationships between customer requirements and services that meet those requirements. This helps ensure that the end product meets the customer's requirements rather than those of the organization.*

SOURCE: *UMMC.*

Step 6. Analyze the organization's strengths and weaknesses

The UMMC QFD team is currently in step 6 of the QFD process. This step is being done in combination with step 7, which measures our competitive positioning. Both are being done through a single survey of our referring physicians. We are asking them to compare the quality of our services with similar services provided at other institutions. This will help us identify who our customers consider to be the top-ranking competitors and measure where we rank relative to competitors.

Future steps

The final phases of the QFD process involve combining the information from steps 4, 5, 6, and 7. Within the matrix, mathematical models enable the team to prioritize areas of improvement. The matrix relationships identified in step 5 are combined with customer requirements (step 4), our own organization's strengths and priorities (step 6), and where we stand relative to our competitors (step 7). This will allow us to determine priorities for change regarding how to enhance services offered.

Results to Date

Through analyzing the voice of the customer, we learned that referring physicians wanted information about new programs given in a letter, rather than in a glossy brochure. This change was made at the launching of a new service. Rather than preparing a brochure, which would have cost $20,000, we prepared a short and focused letter that was distributed to referring physicians. This strategy led to a 14% increase in referral activity over projections. We also learned that referring physicians wanted continuing medical education programs at no cost and in more convenient locations. After applying both strategies, attendance rates tripled, from an average of 50 to an average of 150 to 200 participants per education program. Through these programs, we can enhance referrals as we are better able to assess and meet the specific requirements of our referring physicians.

Conclusion

The QFD process is time-consuming, but worth the investment. Although the MPU team is still in the process of completing the QFD process, valuable lessons have already been learned, and changes have been implemented that have saved significant time and money.

QFD was used because the organization already had a strong committment to TQM. However, QFD has helped strengthen the medical center's paradigm shift, from conducting business as it is most suited to the medical center, to listening to the customer and conducting business to meet customer needs. Instead of assuming that we know what the customer wants, or not asking because we cannot fix it anyway, we now ask questions about what is most important to them. We then use the information to transform the services provided to meet customer needs. Although some information learned may seem self-evident, it has been useful because it has provided data directly from the customer. The QFD process has given validity and emphasis to changes required by the customer.

References

1. Gustafson DH: *Customer needs assessment* (Seminar given at the National Forum on Quality Improvement in Health Care), Orlando, FL, Dec 1992.

2. Gustafson DH, et al: Assessing the needs of breast cancer patients and their families. *Qual Manag Health Care* 2(1): 6–17, Fall 1993.

3. Akao Y, (ed): *Quality Function Deployment: Integrating Customer Requirements into Product Design* trans Glenn Mazur. Cambridge, MA: Productivity Press, 1990.

4. Hauser JR, Clausing D: The house of quality. *Harv Bus Rev* 66(3): 63–73, May/Jun 1988.

5. King B: *Better Designs in Half the Time*, 3rd ed., Methuen, MA: GOAL/QPC, 1989.

Understanding the Patient's Perspective

Appendix A

The "Improving Organizational Performance" Standards from the 1995 AMH

Preamble

This chapter represents a significant evolution in understanding quality improvement in health care organizations. It identifies the connection between organizational performance and judgments about quality. It shifts the primary focus from the performance of individuals to the performance of the organization's systems and processes,* while continuing to recognize the importance of the individual competence of medical staff members and other staff. The **goal** of this improving organizational performance function, then, is that the organization designs processes well and systematically measures, assesses, and improves its performance to improve patient health outcomes. Moreover, this chapter provides flexibility to organizations in how they go about

---

* Throughout the remainder of this chapter, **process** means a single process and/or a system of integrated processes.

their design, measurement, assessment, and improvement activities. Thus, this chapter describes the essential activities common to a wide variety of improvement approaches.

Improving performance has been at the heart of the Joint Commission's Agenda for Change since its inception. This *Accreditation Manual for Hospitals, Volume I (AMH, Vol I)* focuses on the important functions of an organization, and this chapter focuses on a framework for improving those functions. It should now be evident that:

- Performance is *what* is done and *how* well it is done to provide health care.
- The level of performance in health care is
  -the degree to which *what* is done is *efficacious* and *appropriate* for the individual patient; and
  -the degree to which it is *available* in a *timely* manner to patients who need it, *effective, continuous* with other care and care providers, *safe, efficient,* and *caring and respectful* of the patient.

These characteristics of *what* is done and *how well* it is done are called "dimensions of performance."

- The degree to which a hospital does the right things and does them well is influenced strongly by the way it designs and carries out a number of important functions—many of which are described in this *Manual.*

- The effect of an organization's performance of these functions is reflected in patient outcomes and in the cost of its services.

- Patients and others judge the quality of health care based on the patient health outcomes (and sometimes on their perceptions of what was done and how it was done).

- Patients and others may also judge the value of the health care by comparing their judgments about quality with the cost of the health care.

Table 1 page 110, defines dimensions of performance.

This chapter, indeed this entire *Manual*, is being issued at a time when the health care field is redesigning its performance-improvement mechanisms to incorporate concepts and methods developed by other fields. Such concepts and methods include total quality management (TQM), continuous quality improvement (CQI), and systems thinking. The health care field is also incorporating into its performance-improvement mechanisms concepts and methods developed by the health service research community, such as reference databases, clinical practice guidelines or parameters, and functional status and quality-of-life measures. These standards combine many of these useful concepts and methods with the best of current hospital quality assurance activities.

Health care organizations have begun to adopt some of the many approaches to CQI or TQM that have been successful in industry. Most of these approaches give health care organizations' leaders and staff members many powerful methods and tools that are useful additions to those already used in health care. Also, most of these approaches highlight the pivotal role of the organizations' leaders and the importance of assessing patients' needs and expectations and listening to their feedback.

Although the standards in this chapter (as well as elsewhere in this *Manual*) do not require that an organization specifically adopt a CQI or TQM program, they selectively incorporate several core concepts of CQI and TQM. Examples of CQI and TQM concepts in the standards include the key role that leaders (individually and collectively) play in enabling the systematic assessment and improvement of performance; the fact that most problems or opportunities for improvement derive from process weaknesses, not individual incompetence; the need for careful

Table 1. Definitions of Dimensions of Performance

I. Doing the Right Thing

The **efficacy** of the procedure or treatment in relation to the patient's condition

> The degree to which the care of the patient has been shown to accomplish the desired or projected outcome(s)

The **appropriateness** of a specific test, procedure, or service to meet the patient's needs

> The degree to which the care provided is relevant to the patient's clinical needs, given the current state of knowledge

II. Doing the Right Thing Well

The **availability** of a needed test, procedure, treatment, or service to the patient who needs it

> The degree to which appropriate care is available to meet the patient's needs

The **timeliness** with which a needed test, procedure, treatment, or service is provided to the patient

> The degree to which the care is provided to the patient at the most beneficial or necessary time

The **effectiveness** with which tests, procedures, treatments, and services are provided

> The degree to which the care is provided in the correct manner, given the current state of knowledge, to achieve the desired or projected outcome(s) for the patient

The **continuity** of the services provided to the patient with respect to other services, practitioners, and providers and over time

> The degree to which the care for the patient is coordinated among practitioners, among organizations, and over time

The **safety** of the patient (and others) to whom the services are provided

> The degree to which the risk of an intervention and the risk in the care environment are reduced for the patient and others, including the health care provider

The **efficiency** with which services are provided

> The relationship between the outcomes (results of care) and the resources used to deliver patient care

The **respect and caring** with which services are provided

> The degree to which the patient or a designee is involved in his or her own care decisions and to which those providing services do so with sensitivity and respect for the patient's needs, expectations, and individual differences

coordination of work and collaboration among departments and professional groups; the importance of seeking judgments about quality from patients and others and using such judgments to identify areas for improvement; the importance of carefully setting priorities for improvement; and the need for both systematically improving the performance of important functions and maintaining the stability of these functions.

The standards do not require adoption of any particular management style, subscription to any specific "school" of CQI or TQM, use of specific quality improvement tools (for example, Hoshin planning), or adherence to any specific process for improvement (for example, the Joint Commission's "Ten-Step Model").

The standards in this chapter do reflect the need for

- measurement on a continuing basis to understand and maintain the systems and processes (for example, statistical quality control);
- measurement of outcomes to help determine priorities for improving systems and processes; and
- assessment of individual competence and performance (including by peer review), when appropriate.

This chapter has some important links to the other chapters in this *Manual* and, therefore, to other important functions of a health care organization. In particular,

- the chapter presents the performance-improvement framework for use in designing, measuring, assessing, and improving the patient care and organizational functions identified by all the chapters—including this chapter—in this *Manual*. The standards in this chapter point organizations to those functions and processes most directly related to good patient outcomes (PI.3.2 through PI.3.4.2.4) and help organizations set criteria for identifying and prioritizing their improvement efforts.

- the organization's leaders must provide the stimulus, vision, and resources to permit the activities described in this chapter to be successfully implemented. Standards in the "Leadership" chapter identify their role.
- managing the data required to design, measure, assess, and improve patient care and organizational functions requires an organizationwide approach. The standards in the "Management of Information" chapter describe this approach.
- to lead and participate effectively in improvement activities, leaders and staff must acquire the necessary new knowledge. The standards in the "Management of Human Resources" chapter and the "Medical Staff" chapter set the expectations for education and address this continuing knowledge acquisition process.

Finally, the scoring guidelines for this chapter have been designed expressly to help organizations envision the long-term goals of the standards and make progress toward those goals. The activities described in this chapter will take varying periods of time to implement fully, require varying types and levels of change, and may require resource acquisition or reallocation. Thus, expectations for full compliance with many of these standards will be phased into the survey and scoring process at a pace consistent with the field's readiness.

The terms used in this chapter are defined as they are used in the context of the organizational function and may not reflect common dictionary usage.

Definitions

assess To transform data into information by analyzing the data.

criteria Expected level(s) of achievement, or specifications against which performance can be assessed.

improve To take actions that result in the desired measurable change in the identified performance dimension.

indicator A tool used to measure, over time, the performance of functions, processes, and outcomes of an organization.

measure To collect quantifiable data about a dimension of performance, including outcomes, of a function or process.

measurement The systematic process of data collection, repeated over time or at a single point in time.

organizationwide Throughout the organization and across multiple structural and staffing components, as appropriate.

outcome The result of the performance (or nonperformance) of a function or process(es).

performance measure A measure, such as a standard or indicator, used to assess the performance of a function or process of any organization.

plan To formulate or describe the approach to achieving the goals related to improving the performance of the organization.

process A goal-directed, interrelated series of actions, events, mechanisms, or steps.

reference database An organized collection of similar data from many organizations that can be used to compare an organization's performance to that of others.

relevant Having a clearly decisive bearing on an issue.

sentinel event An occurrence that, when noted, requires intensive assessment.

systematic Pursuing a defined objective(s) in a planned, step-by-step manner.

variance A measure of the differences in a set of observations.

variation The differences in results obtained in measuring the same phenomenon more than once. The sources of variation in a process over time can be grouped into two major classes: common causes and special causes.

Plan

If an organization is to initiate and maintain improvement, leadership and planning are essential. This is especially critical for coalescing existing and new improvement activities into a systematic, organizationwide approach. These standards point to the importance of a planned approach to improvement and to the need to have all units (for example, services) and all disciplines (for example, professional groups) collaborating to carry out that approach.

PI.1

The organization has a planned, systematic, organizationwide approach to designing, measuring, assessing, and improving its performance.

PI.1.1 The activities described in this chapter are carried out collaboratively and include the appropriate department(s) and discipline(s) involved.

Design

New processes can be designed well if done systematically and if at least four essential information sources (PI.2.1.1 through PI.2.1.4) are considered that can guide the design process. Each of these sources can identify design specifications and expectations against which success can be measured.

PI.2

New processes are designed well.

PI.2.1 The design is based on

    PI.2.1.1 the organization's mission, vision, and plans;

    PI.2.1.2 the needs and expectations of patients, staff, and others;

    PI.2.1.3 up-to-date sources of information about designing processes (such as practice guidelines or parameters); and

    PI.2.1.4 the performance of the processes and their outcomes in other organizations (such as information from reference databases).

Measure

Measurement, (that is, the collection of data) is the basis for determining the level of performance of existing processes and the outcomes resulting from these processes. To provide useful data, measurement must be systematic, relate to relevant dimensions of performance, and be of appropriate breadth and frequency.

The standards in this section address issues such as the purposes of measurement, the selection crieria for functions, processes and outcomes to be measured, the important sources of data, and the continued role of measuring.

PI.3

The organization has in place a systematic process to collect data needed to

- design and assess new processes;
- assess the dimensions of performance relevant to functions, processes, and outcomes;
- measure the level of performance and stability* of important existing processes;
- identify areas for possible improvement of existing processes; and
- determine whether changes improved the processes.

PI.3.1 The collected data include measures of both processes and outcomes.

PI.3.2 Data are collected both for the priority issues chosen for improvement and as part of continuing measurement.

PI.3.3 The organization collects data about

PI.3.3.1 the needs and expectations of patients and others and the degree to which these needs and expectations have been met; and

---

* A stable process can have very large common-cause variation. So it is possible to have a process that is stable, yet incapable of performing satisfactorily.

PI.3.3.1.1 These data relate to the relevant dimensions of performance.

PI.3.3.2 its staff's views regarding current performance and opportunities for improvement.

PI.3.4 The organization measures the performance of processes in all the patient care and organizational functions identified in this Manual.

PI.3.4.1 Processes measured on a continuing basis include those that

PI.3.4.1.1 affect a large percentage of patients; and/or

PI.3.4.1.2 place patients at serious risk if not performed well, or performed when not indicated, or not performed when indicated; and/or

PI.3.4.1.3 have been or are likely to be problem prone.

PI.3.4.2 Processes measured encompass at least

PI.3.4.2.1 those related to use of operative and other invasive procedures, including (1) selecting appropriate procedures, (2) preparing the patient for the procedure, (3) performing the procedure and monitoring the patient, and (4) providing postprocedure care;

PI.3.4.2.2 those related to the use of medications, including (1) prescribing or ordering medication, (2) preparing and dispensing, (3) administration, and (4) monitoring the medications' effects on patients;

PI.3.4.2.3 those related to use of blood and blood components, including (1) ordering, (2) distributing, handling, and dispensing, (3) administration, and (4) monitoring the blood and blood components' effects on patients; and

PI.3.4.2.4 those related to determining the appropriateness of admissions and continued hospitalization (that is, utilization-management activities).

PI.3.5 The organization collects data about

PI.3.5.1 autopsy results;

PI.3.5.2 risk-management activities; and

PI.3.5.3 quality-control activities in at least the following areas:

PI.3.5.3.1 Clinical laboratory services,

PI.3.5.3.2 Diagnostic radiology services,

PI.3.5.3.3 Dietetic services,

PI.3.5.3.4 Nuclear medicine services, and

PI.3.5.3.5 Radiation oncology services.

Assess

Interpretation of the collected data provides information about the organization's level of performance along many dimenstions and over time. Assessment questions include, for example,

- What is the degree of conformance to process and outcome objectives?
- How stable is a process, or how consistent is an outcome?
- Where might a stable process be improved?
- Was the indesirable variation in a process or outcome reduced or eliminated?

In addition to assessing performance over time, further information is gained from comparing data among organizations when relevant databases exist.

The standards in this section address the elements of a systematic assessment process and emphasize the importance of asking the right assessment questions and using the right processes and mechanisms to answer these questions.

PI.4

The organization has a systematic process to assess collected data in order to determine

- whether design specifications for new processes were met;
- the level of performance and stability of important existing processes;
- priorities for possible improvement of existing processes;

- actions to improve the performance of processes; and
- whether changes in the processes resulted in improvement.

PI.4.1 The assessment process includes

    PI.4.1.1 using statistical quality control techniques, as appropriate;

    PI.4.1.2 comparing data about

        PI.4.1.2.1 the organization's processes and outcomes over time,

        PI.4.1.2.2 the organization's processes to the information from up-to-date sources about the design and performance of processes (such as practice guidelines or parameters), and

        PI.4.1.2.3 the organization's performance of processes and their outcomes to that of other organizations, including using reference databases; and

    PI.4.1.3 intensive assessment when undesirable variation in performance may have occurred or is occurring. Such intensive assessments are initiated

        PI.4.1.3.1 by important single events and by absolute levels and/or patterns or trends that significantly and undesirably vary from those expected, based on appropriate statistical analysis;

        PI.4.1.3.2 when the organization's performance significantly and undesirably varies from that of other organizations;

        PI.4.1.3.3 when the organization's performance significantly and undesirably varies from recognized standards;

        PI.4.1.3.4 when the organization wishes to improve already good performance;

        PI.4.1.3.5 Intensive assessment when undesirable variation in performance may have occurred or is occurring. Such intensive assessments are initiated in response to all major discrepancies, or patterns of discrepancies, between preoperative and postoperative (including pathologic) diagnoses, including those identified during the pathologic review of specimens removed during operative or invasive procedures;

PI.4.1.3.6 by all confirmed transfusion reactions; and

PI.4.1.3.7 by all significant adverse drug reactions.

PI.4.2 When the findings of the assessment process are relevant to an individual's performance,

PI.4.2.1 the medical staff is responsible for determining their use in peer review and/or the periodic evaluations of a licensed independent practitioner's competence, in accordance with the standards on renewing and revising clinical privileges in the "Medical Staff" chapter (MS.4.3.3); and/or

PI.4.2.2 the service director is responsible for determining the competence of individuals who are not licensed independent practitioners, in accordance with LD.2.1.5 and HR.4.

Improve

The activities described in PI.3 will identify a variety of opportunities for improvement. These include

- designing new processes and/or reducing variation or eleminating undesirable variation in processes or outcomes; and

- improving already well-performing existing processes.

The standards in this section address the elements of a systematic approach to improvement: planning the change, testing it, studying its effect, and implementing changes that are worthwhile improvements.

PI.5.1 The organization systematically improves its performance.

PI.5.1 Existing processes are improved when an organization decides to act on an opportunity for improvement or when the measurement of an existing process identifies that an undesirable change in performance may have occurred or is occurring.

PI.5.1.1 These decisions consider

PI.5.1.1.1 opportunities to improve processes within the important functions described in this *Manual*;

PI.5.1.1.2 the factors listed in PI.3.3 through PI.3.5.3.5;

PI.5.1.1.3 the resources required to make the improvement; and

PI.5.1.1.4 the organization's mission and priorities.

PI.5.2 The design or improvement activities

PI.5.2.1 specifically consider the expected impact of the design or improvement on the relevant dimensions of performance;

PI.5.2.2 set performance expectations for the newly designed or

improved processes;

PI.5.2.3 include adopting, adapting, or creating measures of the performance; and

PI.5.2.4 involve those individuals, professions, and services closest to the design or improvement activity.

PI.5.3 The primary focus of design or improvement activities is on those processes that need to be improved and include

PI.5.3.1 planning the action;

PI.5.3.1.1 When the plan includes testing on a trial basis, new actions are planned when tested actions are not effective.

PI.5.3.2 measuring and assessing the effect of the action; and

PI.5.3.3 implementing effective actions.

PI.5.3.3.1 Pursuant to PI.4.2, when improvement activities lead to a determination that an individual has performance problems that he or she is unable or unwilling to improve, his or her clinical privileges or job assignment are modified, as indicated, or other appropriate action is taken (in accordance with the standards on renewing and revising clinical privileges in the "Medical Staff" chapter and on determining competence in the "Management of Human Resources" chapter).

Understanding the Patient's Perspective

Appendix B

Additional Resources

The following list of articles and books is intended to provide readers with additional information on the topics discussed in this publication.

Research on Patient Needs and Satisfaction

Cleary PD, McNeil BJ: Patient satisfaction as an indicator of quality care. *Inquiry* 25 (1): 25–36, Spring 1988.

Cleary PD, et al: Patients evaluate their hospital care: A national survey. *Health Aff* 10 (4): 254–267, Winter 1991.

Davies AR, Ware JE, Jr: Involving consumers in quality of care assessment: Do they provide valid information? *Health Aff* 7(1) 33–48, Spring 1988.

Donabedian A: The quality of care: How can it be assessed? JAMA 260(12): 1743–1748, Sep 1988.

Hulka BS, et al: Correlates of satisfaction and dissatisfaction with medical care: A community perspective. *Med Care* 13(8): 648–658, Aug 1975.

Lebow JL: Consumer assessments of the quality of medical care. *Med Care* 12(4): 328–337, Apr 1974.

Linder-Pelz S: Social psychological determinants of patient satisfaction: A test of five hypotheses. *Soc Sci Medicine* 16(5): 583–589, 1982.

Linn LS: Factors associated with patient evaluation of health care. *Milbank Mem Fund Q Health Soc* 53(4): 531–548, Fall 1975.

Linn LS, Greenfield S: Patient suffering and patient satisfaction among the chronically ill. *Med Care* 20(4): 425–431, Apr 1982.

Nelson EC, et al: The patient judgment system: Reliability and validity. *QRB* 15(6): 185–191, Jun 1989.

Pascoe GC: Patient satisfaction in primary health care: A literature review and analysis. *Eval Prog Plann* 6(3–4): 185, 1983.

Press I, Ganey R: Quality of care and patient satisfaction. *The Quality Letter for Healthcare Leaders* 2(1): 11–13, Feb 1990.

Strasser S, et al: The patient satisfaction process: Moving toward a comprehensive model. *Med Care Rev* 50(2): 219–248, Summer 1993.

Swan J: Deepening the understanding of hospital patient satisfaction: Fulfillment and equity effects. *Journal of Health Care Marketing* 5(13): 7–18, Summer 1983.

Tarlov AR, et al: The medical outcomes study: An application of methods for monitoring the results of medical care. *JAMA* 262(7): 925, Aug 1989.

Ware JE, et al: Consumer perceptions of health care services: Implications for academic medicine. *J Med Educ* 50(9): 839–848, Sep 1975.

Ware JE, et al: The measurement and meaning of patient satisfaction. *Health and Medical Care Service Review* 1(1): 3–5, Jan/Feb 1978.

Wartman SA, et al: Patient understanding and satisfaction as predictor of compliance. *Med Care* 21(9): 886–891, Sep 1983.

Tying Feedback to Quality Improvement

Batalden PB, Nelson EC: Hospital quality: Patient, physician and employee judgments. *International Journal of Health Care Quality Assurance* 3(4): 7–17, 1990.

Batalden PB, Nelson EC: Patient-based quality measurement systems. *Quality Management in Health Care* 2(1): 18–30, Fall 1993.

Deming WE: *Out of the Crisis.* Cambridge, MA: Massachusetts Institute of Technology Press, 1986.

Gerteis M: *Through the Patient's Eyes. Understanding and Promoting Patient-Centered Care.* San Francisco, CA: Jossey-Bass Publishers, 1993.

Gustafson DH, et al: Assessing the needs of breast cancer patients and their families. *Quality Management in Health Care* 2(1): 6–17, Fall 1993.

Harper Peterson MB: Measuring patient satisfaction: Collecting useful data. *J Nurs Qual Assur* 2(3): 26, May 1988.

Juran JM: *Juran on Planning for Quality*. New York: The Free Press, 1988.

Kano SN, et al: *Attractive Quality and Must-Be Quality*. Methuen, MA: GOAL/QPC, 1984.

King B: *Better Designs in Half the Time: Implementing QFD Quality Function Deployment in America*, 3rd ed. Methuen, MA: GOAL/QPC, 1989.

Koska MT: Surveying customer needs, not satisfaction, is crucial to CQI. *Hospitals* 66(21): 50–53, Nov 1992.

Moen RD, et al: *Improving Quality Through Planned Experimentation*. New York: McGraw-Hill, 1991.

Nelson EC, et al: Gaining customer knowledge: Obtaining and using customer judgments for hospitalwide quality improvement. *Top Health Rec Manage* 11(3): 13–26, Mar 1991.

Owad WP, Jr: Developing a customer-driven approach to quality improvement systems. *Top Hosp Pharm Manage* 12(4): 8–68, Jan 1993.

Strasser S, Davis RM: *Measuring Patient Satisfaction for Improved Patient Services*. Ann Arbor, MI: Health Administration Press, 1991.

Waggoner DM: Application of continuous quality improvement techniques to the treatment of patients with hypertension. *Health Care Manage Rev* 17(3): 33–42, Summer 1992.

Research Methods

Fink A, Kosecoff J: *How To Conduct Surveys. A Step-by-Step Guide*. Newbury Park, CA: Sage Publications, 1985.

Fowler FJ, Jr: *Survey Research Methods*. Newbury Park, CA: Sage Publications, 1988.

Frey JH: *Survey Research by Telephone*, 2nd ed. Newbury Park, CA: Sage Publications, 1989.

Henry G: *Practical Sampling*. Newbury Park, CA: Sage Publications, 1990.

Ishikawa K: *Guide to Quality Control*. White Plains: Kraus International Publications, 1982.

Kidder L, Judd C: *Research Methods in Social Relations*. Fort Worth, TX: Holt, Rinehart and Winston, 1990.

Lipsey M: *Design Sensitivity*. Newbury Park, CA: Sage Publications, 1990.

Payne SL: *The Art of Asking Questions*. Princeton, NJ: Princeton University Press, 1951.

Quinn D: Principles of data collection applied to customer knowledge. *J Healthc Qual* 14(6): 24–36, Nov/Dec 1992.

Stewart D, Shamdasani P: *Focus Groups: Theory and Practice*. Newbury Park, CA: Sage Publications, 1990.

Steiber SR, Krowinski WJ: *Measuring and Managing Patient Satisfaction*. Chicago: American Hospital Association Publishing, 1990.

Tufte ER: *The Visual Display of Quantitative Information*. Cheshire, CT: Graphics Press, 1983.

Appendix C

Needs Assessment Surveys

Survey of Information Needs about Breast Cancer

This study has been planned to identify the information needs of women who have been diagnosed with breast cancer. We will use the results to develop programs to help these women with breast cancer and their families. We are asking you to help us identify the most important types of information *needed right after learning about the breast cancer*.

We would like you to fill out the following survey. It should take no more than 40 minutes of your time. We will not ask you to include your name with your answers. This means your answers will be anonymous. No one will be able to know which answers were yours. Please be honest in answering the questions.

Whether or not you want to answer these questions is up to you. You do not have to participate. Also, you may choose not to finish the survey. Deciding not to answer the questions will not affect your present or future medical care. If you return a completed questionnaire, we will assume you have chosen to participate in the study.

If you have questions about this research, please do not hesitate to contact:

©Center for Health Systems Research and Analysis 1991
Version II - May 14, 1991
University of Wisconsin - Madison
David Gustafson (608) 293-0492

For the following questions, please check the box corresponding to the importance of the information to you.

	Not Important	Slightly Important	Important	Very Important	Essential

1. GENERAL INFORMATION

	Not Important	Slightly Important	Important	Very Important	Essential
A Explanations of technical/medical terms	❑	❑	❑	❑	❑
B Lists of articles about breast cancer	❑	❑	❑	❑	❑
C Easy to understand summaries of breast cancer studies	❑	❑	❑	❑	❑
D Current statistics on breast cancer	❑	❑	❑	❑	❑
E Questions to ask a doctor about breast cancer	❑	❑	❑	❑	❑
F How to find someone to give me information	❑	❑	❑	❑	❑
G What causes breast cancer	❑	❑	❑	❑	❑

2. REFERRAL

	Not Important	Slightly Important	Important	Very Important	Essential
A How to find someone for support/advice	❑	❑	❑	❑	❑
B How to choose a doctor (what criteria?)	❑	❑	❑	❑	❑
C Right to switch doctors	❑	❑	❑	❑	❑
D How to switch doctors	❑	❑	❑	❑	❑
E Right not to follow doctor's recommendations	❑	❑	❑	❑	❑
F How to tell a doctor if you don't agree with recommendations	❑	❑	❑	❑	❑
G Where the most up-to-date medicine is practiced	❑	❑	❑	❑	❑
H How to find the religious support one needs	❑	❑	❑	❑	❑

3. EARLY DETECTION

	Not Important	Slightly Important	Important	Very Important	Essential
A Having a program available that promotes regular professional and self-exam	❑	❑	❑	❑	❑
B Training on how to examine breasts and interpret changes	❑	❑	❑	❑	❑

4. DIAGNOSIS

	Not Important	Slightly Important	Important	Very Important	Essential
A What the diagnosis of breast cancer really means to me	❑	❑	❑	❑	❑
B How much time is reasonable between diagnosis and treatment	❑	❑	❑	❑	❑

	Not Important	Slightly Important	Important	Very Important	Essential
C What questions the doctors may ask and why they will ask them	❏	❏	❏	❏	❏
D What questions you as a patient may want to ask	❏	❏	❏	❏	❏

5. PROSPECT OF RECOVERY

A What factors influence the recovery process?	❏	❏	❏	❏	❏
B What does the future hold (hair loss, change in lifestyle, change in sexuality)?	❏	❏	❏	❏	❏
C What are the chances of another cancer developing?	❏	❏	❏	❏	❏

6. TREATMENT (WHAT IT IS, EFFECTIVENESS, AND SIDE EFFECTS)

A Surgery	❏	❏	❏	❏	❏
B Radiotherapy	❏	❏	❏	❏	❏
C Tamoxifen (Nolvadex)	❏	❏	❏	❏	❏
D Chemotherapy	❏	❏	❏	❏	❏
E Nontraditional treatments	❏	❏	❏	❏	❏

7. HELP WITH DECISIONS

A Mastectomy vs lumpectomy (surgery that would not take the whole breast)	❏	❏	❏	❏	❏
B Chemotherapy or hormonal treatment (or both)	❏	❏	❏	❏	❏
C Reconstruction of breast or prosthesis (artificial breast)	❏	❏	❏	❏	❏
D How to take control of my decision	❏	❏	❏	❏	❏

8. REHABILITATION

A Exercises (explanation of and training in)	❏	❏	❏	❏	❏
B Time required to recover physically	❏	❏	❏	❏	❏
C How far will you come back to the way you were before physically?	❏	❏	❏	❏	❏
D What symptoms are normal during recovery?	❏	❏	❏	❏	❏

	Not Important	Slightly Important	Important	Very Important	Essential

9. INTERACTIONS

A How to counsel people who have breast changes or cancer (what to say/not to say)   ❑   ❑   ❑   ❑   ❑

B How to talk openly about my breast changes/cancer with friends and family   ❑   ❑   ❑   ❑   ❑

C How to communicate to people what I'm going through   ❑   ❑   ❑   ❑   ❑

D How, what, when, whether, and why to tell a particular person about my breast problems   ❑   ❑   ❑   ❑   ❑

E How to find a support group, what to do if no support group is in town or nearby   ❑   ❑   ❑   ❑   ❑

F How my family/friends and I can support each other   ❑   ❑   ❑   ❑   ❑

G How to deal with friends who don't support me   ❑   ❑   ❑   ❑   ❑

H How to get past my doctor's tough exterior   ❑   ❑   ❑   ❑   ❑

10. SEXUALITY

A What are the effects of chemotherapy and tamoxifen (Nolvadex) on sexual activity (not only intercourse)?   ❑   ❑   ❑   ❑   ❑

B When is it safe to have intercourse?   ❑   ❑   ❑   ❑   ❑

C How to deal with any guilt over not wanting intercourse, and saying "no" to it   ❑   ❑   ❑   ❑   ❑

D How to deal with constantly thinking about breasts after I have lost one   ❑   ❑   ❑   ❑   ❑

E How to deal with my body image   ❑   ❑   ❑   ❑   ❑

F How/when to tell a new partner about previous mastectomy and problems with breast   ❑   ❑   ❑   ❑   ❑

G Will my treatment affect the health of any children that I might have in the future?   ❑   ❑   ❑   ❑   ❑

	Not Important	Slightly Important	Important	Very Important	Essential

11. COPING WITH

A Living with uncertainty (dealing with fears and lack of answers to questions)	❑	❑	❑	❑	❑
B Coming to terms with the possibility of death	❑	❑	❑	❑	❑
C Loss of youth, future, changing, dealing with what "I will and won't be able to do"	❑	❑	❑	❑	❑
D Making sure that spouse/partner doesn't feel shut out	❑	❑	❑	❑	❑
E How to deal with children's reactions	❑	❑	❑	❑	❑
F Coping with physical reactions to treatment	❑	❑	❑	❑	❑
G Answering the question "Why me?"	❑	❑	❑	❑	❑
H Dealing with any guilt (from saying "no" to chemotherapy to not having a positive attitude)	❑	❑	❑	❑	❑

12. FINANCES

A What should a good insurance policy cover?	❑	❑	❑	❑	❑
B Will my insurance or employer cover the costs, and what can I do if they don't?	❑	❑	❑	❑	❑
C How can I get special surgeries paid for (nipple surgery, etc)?	❑	❑	❑	❑	❑
D What can I do if doctors' charges are unreasonable or for more than the insurance will pay?	❑	❑	❑	❑	❑
E Can I get the insurance company to let me go to an outside provider? If so, how?	❑	❑	❑	❑	❑
F What can I do about switching insurance with preexisting conditions?	❑	❑	❑	❑	❑
G Do I have rights to Social Security Disability?	❑	❑	❑	❑	❑

	Not Important	Slightly Important	Important	Very Important	Essential
H What are my rights for medical leave from work?	❑	❑	❑	❑	❑
I What can I do if my rights are abused?	❑	❑	❑	❑	❑

13. TRANSITIONS

	Not Important	Slightly Important	Important	Very Important	Essential
A Knowledge of what happens between:					
(a) diagnosis and surgery	❑	❑	❑	❑	❑
(b) surgery and radiotherapy	❑	❑	❑	❑	❑
(c) surgery and chemotherapy	❑	❑	❑	❑	❑
(d) chemotherapy and radiation	❑	❑	❑	❑	❑
B How to deal with new people/ practitioners in the next stage of treatment	❑	❑	❑	❑	❑
C What ties will I maintain with my previous doctor and how can I maintain these ties?	❑	❑	❑	❑	❑
D Who will be my next doctor and what is s/he like?	❑	❑	❑	❑	❑

14. Please list the most important questions and concerns you have about breast cancer today:

_____

_____

_____

_____

_____

_____

_____

In this section, we ask you for your views on *your health*.

Please answer each question by marking the appropriate box.
If you are unsure abut how to answer a question. please give the best answer you can.

(Questions 15 to 25 used by permission. Copyright New England Medical Center, 1990. All Rights Reserved.)

15. In general, would you say your health is:

❑ Excellent   ❑ Good   ❑ Poor
❑ Very Good   ❑ Fair

16. *Compared to 4 weeks ago,* how would you rate your health in general now?

❑ Much better than 4 weeks ago
❑ Somewhat better than 4 weeks ago
❑ About the same
❑ Somewhat worse than 4 weeks ago

17. The following questions are about activities you might do during a typical day. Does your health now limit these activities? Is so, how much? (Check one box for each line.)

	Yes, limited a lot	Yes, limited a little	No, not limited at all
A *Vigorous activities*, such as running, lifting heavy objects, participating in strenuous sports	❑	❑	❑
B *Moderate activities*, such as moving a table, pushing a vacuum cleaner, bowling, or playing golf	❑	❑	❑
C Lifting or carrying groceries	❑	❑	❑
D Climbing *several* flights of stairs	❑	❑	❑
E Climbing *one* flight of stairs	❑	❑	❑
F Bending, kneeling, or stooping	❑	❑	❑
G Walking more *than a mile*	❑	❑	❑
H Walking *several blocks*	❑	❑	❑
I Walking *one block*	❑	❑	❑
J Bathing or dressing yourself	❑	❑	❑

18. During the *past 2 weeks*, have you had any of the following problems with your work or other regular daily activities *as a result of your physical health?* (Check one box for each line.)

	Yes	No
A Cut down the *amount of time* you spent on work or other activities	❑	❑
B *Accomplished less* than you would like	❑	❑
C Were limited in the *kind* of work or other activities	❑	❑
D Had *difficulty* performing the work or other activities (for example, it took extra effort)	❑	❑

19. During the *past 2 weeks*, have you had any of the following problems with your work or other regular daily activities *as a result of any emotional problems* (such as feeling depressed or anxious)? (Check one box for each line.)

	Yes	No
A Cut down the *amount of time* you spent on work or other activities	❑	❑
B *Accomplished less* than you would like	❑	❑
C Didn't do work or other activities as *carefully* as usual	❑	❑

20. During the *past 2 weeks*, to what extent has your physical health or emotional problems interfered with your normal social activities with family, friends, neighbors, or groups? (Check one box.)

❑ Not at all   ❑ Quite a bit
❑ Slightly   ❑ Extremely
❑ Modeerately

21. How much bodily pain have you had during the *past 2 weeks?* (Check one box.)

❑ None   ❑ Moderate
❑ Very Mild   ❑ Severe
❑ Mild   ❑ Very severe

22. During the *past 2 weeks*, how much did pain interfere with your normal work (including both work outside the home and housework)? (Check one box.)

❑ Not at all   ❑ Quite a bit
❑ A little bit   ❑ Extremely
❑ Moderately

23. These questions are about how you feel and how things have been with you during the *past 2 weeks*. For each question, please give the one answer that comes closest to the way you have been feeling. How much during the *past 2 weeks* . . . (Mark one box on each line.)

	All of the time	Most of the time	Good amount of the time	Mostly false	Definitely false
A Did you feel peppy?	❏	❏	❏	❏	❏
B Have you been a very nervous person?	❏	❏	❏	❏	❏
C Have you felt so down in the dumps nothing could cheer you up?	❏	❏	❏	❏	❏
D Have you felt calm and peaceful?	❏	❏	❏	❏	❏
E Did you have a lot of energy?	❏	❏	❏	❏	❏
F Have you felt downhearted and blue?	❏	❏	❏	❏	❏
G Did you feel worn out?	❏	❏	❏	❏	❏
H Have you been a happy person?	❏	❏	❏	❏	❏
I Did you feel tired?	❏	❏	❏	❏	❏

24. During the *past 2 weeks*, how much of the time has your *physical health or emotional problems* interfered with your social activities (like visiting with friends, relatives, etc)?

❏ All of the time   ❏ A little of the time
❏ Most of the time   ❏ None of the time
❏ Some of the time

25. Please choose the answer the best describes how *true or false* each of the following statements is for you. (Check one box for each line.)

	Definitely true	Mostly true	Not sure	Mostly false	Definitely false
A I seem to get sick a little easier than other people	❏	❏	❏	❏	❏
B I am as healthy as anybody I know	❏	❏	❏	❏	❏
C I expect my health to get worse	❏	❏	❏	❏	❏
D My health is excellent	❏	❏	❏	❏	❏

Finally, let us know a little about you.

26. Your age:_____   27. Today's Date   /   /

28. Racial Heritage:
- ❏ African American   ❏ Asian
- ❏ Caucasian   ❏ Hispanic
- ❏ Native American
- ❏ Other

29. Years of schooling that you have had:_____

30. What kind of health insurance do you have? (Check one box.)
- ❏ HMO
- ❏ Medicare/Medicaid
- ❏ Other_____

31. Are you currently employed?   ❏ Yes _____hrs/week   ❏ No

32. When did you learn about your breast cancer?

33. What stage of breast cancer did you have?
- ❏ Stage I   ❏ Stage IV
- ❏ Stage II   ❏ Recurrent
- ❏ Stage III   ❏ Don't Know

34. Please check the treatments that you have had. Write in the approximate date you completed each treatment.

	Date
❏ Surgery	/ /
❏ Reconstruction	/ /
❏ Radiation	/ /
❏ Tamoxifen (Nolvadex)	/ /
❏ Chemotherapy	/ /

35. Please indicate the current stage of your treatment or recovery and, when appropriate, the corresponding date you started.

	Date started
❏ Waiting for surgery	/ /
❏ In radiation treatment	/ /
❏ In chemotherapy	/ /
❏ Recovering from treatment	/ /
❏ Recovery completed	
❏ Other, please specify_____	

THANK YOU AGAIN

Hospitalwide Patient Satisfaction Survey

Please answer this questionnaire for your most recent stay in our hospital. For each question, "X" one box that best answers the question.

BACKGROUND ON YOUR HOSPITAL STAY

1. Before this hospitalization, about how many times have you been admitted to this same hospital and stayed one or more nights?

❏ 1 Never, this was the first time ever
❏ 2 One other time
❏ 3 Two other times
❏ 4 Three or more other times

2. Have you ever been treated before at this hospital as an outpatient or an emergency room patient?

❏ 1 Yes
❏ 2 No

3. Thinking about your recent hospitalization, who chose this hospital? ("X" all that apply. You may choose more than one.)

❏ 1 Doctor chose
❏ 2 Patient or family member chose
❏ 3 Someone else chose
❏ 4 My insurance/health plan requires it

4. Were you admitted to the hospital . . .

❏ 1 Through the Outpatient Department
❏ 2 Through the Admitting Office
❏ 3 Other (Specify)

5. The time it took to get you settled in your room was . . .

❏ 1 Excellent
❏ 2 Very Good
❏ 3 Good
❏ 4 Fair
❏ 5 Poor

6. For *most* of your stay, were you . . .

❏ 1 Alone in a private room
❏ 2 Alone in a semi-private room
❏ 3 In a room with other patient(s)

7. For most of your stay, were you on a special diet or could you *eat regular foods*?

❏ 1 Regular or unrestricted diet
❏ 2 Liquid diet
❏ 3 Special diet
❏ 4 Don't know

8. During your hospital stay, how much help did you need with your everyday activities (eating, bathing, dressing, using the bathroom, getting out of bed)? Did you need . . .

❏ 1 A lot of help
❏ 2 Quite a bit of help
❏ 3 Some help
❏ 4 Little help
❏ 5 Never needed help

9. During your hospital stay, how much pain did you experience?

❏ 1 A lot of pain
❏ 2 Quite a bit of pain
❏ 3 Some pain
❏ 4 A little pain
❏ 5 No pain at all

10. Do you think that the amount of time you spent in the hospital was . . .

❏ 1 About right
❏ 2 Too short
❏ 3 Too long
❏ 4 Not sure

11. Where did you (the patient) stay in the hospital? In a section of the hospital for . . . ("X" all that apply. You may choose more than one.)

❏ 1 Adult surgery only
❏ 2 Adult nonsurgery only
❏ 3 Adult surgery and nonsurgery patients combined together
❏ 4 Heart/Coronary care
❏ 5 Intensive/Critical care
❏ 6 Childbirth/Maternity
❏ 7 Children/Pediatrics (not newborns)
❏ 8 Other (Specify):_____
❏ 9 Can't recall type of unit

Now, we would like you to rate some things about your hospital stay in terms of whether they were *Excellent*, *Very Good*, *Fair*, or *Poor*. Please mark only one answer for each statement. If something does not apply to you, mark *Doesn't apply*.

	Excellent	Very good	Good	Fair	Poor	Doesn't apply

ADMISSION: ENTERING THE HOSPITAL

12. EFFICIENCY OF THE ADMITTING PROCEDURE: Ease of getting admitted, including the amount of time it took

| | ❏ | ❏ | ❏ | ❏ | ❏ | ❏ |

13. PREPARATION FOR ADMISSION: How clear and complete information was about how to prepare for your stay in the hospital and what to expect once you got there

| | ❏ | ❏ | ❏ | ❏ | ❏ | ❏ |

14. ATTENTION OF ADMITTING STAFF TO YOUR INDIVIDUAL NEEDS: Their handling of your personal needs and wants

| | ❏ | ❏ | ❏ | ❏ | ❏ | ❏ |

YOUR DAILY CARE IN THE HOSPITAL

15. CONSIDERATION OF YOUR NEEDS: Willingness of hospital staff to meet your needs

| | ❏ | ❏ | ❏ | ❏ | ❏ | ❏ |

16. COORDINATION OF CARE: The teamwork of all the hospital staff who took care of you

| | ❏ | ❏ | ❏ | ❏ | ❏ | ❏ |

17. HELPFULNESS AND CHEERFULNESS: Ability of hospital staff to make you comfortable and reassure you

| | ❏ | ❏ | ❏ | ❏ | ❏ | ❏ |

18. SENSITIVITY TO PROBLEMS: Sensitivity of hospital staff to your special problems or concerns

| | ❏ | ❏ | ❏ | ❏ | ❏ | ❏ |

	Excellent	Very good	Good	Fair	Poor	Doesn't apply

KEEPING YOU INFORMED

19. EASE OF GETTING INFORMATION: Willingness of hospital staff to answer your questions

| ❑ | ❑ | ❑ | ❑ | ❑ | ❑ |

20. INSTRUCTIONS: How well nurses and other staff explained tests, treatments, and what to expect

| ❑ | ❑ | ❑ | ❑ | ❑ | ❑ |

21. INFORMING FAMILY OR FRIENDS: How well they were kept informed about your condition and needs

| ❑ | ❑ | ❑ | ❑ | ❑ | ❑ |

22. SKILL OF NURSES: How well things were done, like giving medicine and handling IVs

| ❑ | ❑ | ❑ | ❑ | ❑ | ❑ |

23. ATTENTION OF NURSES TO YOUR CONDITION: How often nurses checked on you to keep track of how you were doing

| ❑ | ❑ | ❑ | ❑ | ❑ | ❑ |

24. NURSING STAFF RESPONSE TO YOUR CALLS: How quick they were to help

| ❑ | ❑ | ❑ | ❑ | ❑ | ❑ |

25. CONCERN AND CARING BY NURSES: Courtesy and respect you were given; friendliness and kindness

| ❑ | ❑ | ❑ | ❑ | ❑ | ❑ |

26. INFORMATION GIVEN BY NURSES: How well nurses communicated with patients, families, and doctors

| ❑ | ❑ | ❑ | ❑ | ❑ | ❑ |

YOUR DOCTOR

27. ATTENTION OF DOCTOR TO YOUR CONDITION: How often doctors checked on you to keep track of how you were doing

| ❑ | ❑ | ❑ | ❑ | ❑ | ❑ |

	Excellent	Very good	Good	Fair	Poor	Doesn't apply
28. AVAILABILITY OF DOCTOR: How easy it was to get your doctor when needed	❏	❏	❏	❏	❏	❏
29. CONCERN AND CARING BY DOCTORS: Courtesy and respect you were given; friendliness and kindness	❏	❏	❏	❏	❏	❏
30. SKILL OF DOCTORS: Ability to diagnose problems, thoroughness of examination, and skill in treating your condition	❏	❏	❏	❏	❏	❏
31. INFORMATION GIVEN BY DOCTORS: Amount of information you were given about your illness and treatment; what to do after leaving the hospital	❏	❏	❏	❏	❏	❏
32. COORDINATION: Teamwork among all the doctors who cared for you	❏	❏	❏	❏	❏	❏

OTHER HOSPITAL STAFF

33. HOUSEKEEPING STAFF: How well did they did their jobs and how they acted toward you	❏	❏	❏	❏	❏	❏
34. LABORATORY STAFF: How well they did their jobs and how they acted toward you	❏	❏	❏	❏	❏	❏
35. X-RAY STAFF: How well they did their jobs and how they acted toward you	❏	❏	❏	❏	❏	❏
36. PHYSICAL THERAPY STAFF: How well they did their jobs and how they acted toward you	❏	❏	❏	❏	❏	❏
37. TRANSPORTATION STAFF: How well they did their jobs and how they acted toward you	❏	❏	❏	❏	❏	❏
38. IV STARTER: Skill of staff who started your IV	❏	❏	❏	❏	❏	❏

	Excellent	Very good	Good	Fair	Poor	Doesn't apply

LIVING ARRANGEMENTS

39. PRIVACY: Provisions for your privacy ❏ ❏ ❏ ❏ ❏ ❏

40. CONDITION OF YOUR ROOM: Cleanliness, comfort, lighting, and temperature ❏ ❏ ❏ ❏ ❏ ❏

41. SUPPLIES AND FURNISHINGS: Completeness of supplies provided for your use, condition of the furniture, and how well things worked ❏ ❏ ❏ ❏ ❏ ❏

42. RESTFULNESS OF ATMOSPHERE: Amount of peace and quiet ❏ ❏ ❏ ❏ ❏ ❏

43. QUALITY OF FOOD: Overall, how good it tasted, serving temperature, and variety available ❏ ❏ ❏ ❏ ❏ ❏

44. SIGNS AND DIRECTIONS: Ease of finding your way around the hospital ❏ ❏ ❏ ❏ ❏ ❏

45. HOSPITAL BUILDING: How you would rate the hospital building overall ❏ ❏ ❏ ❏ ❏ ❏

46. PARKING: Number of spaces available, convenience of location, and cost ❏ ❏ ❏ ❏ ❏ ❏

47. PROVISIONS FOR FAMILY AND FRIENDS: Adequacy of visiting hours and facilities for them; visitors treated like welcome guests ❏ ❏ ❏ ❏ ❏ ❏

	Excellent	Very good	Good	Fair	Poor	Doesn't apply

DISCHARGE: LEAVING THE HOSPITAL

48. DISCHARGE PROCEDURES: Time it took to be discharged from the hospital and how efficiently it was handled

❏ ❏ ❏ ❏ ❏ ❏

49. DISCHARGE INSTRUCTIONS: How clearly and completely you were told what to do and what to expect when you left the hospital

❏ ❏ ❏ ❏ ❏ ❏

50. COORDINATION OF CARE AFTER DISCHARGE: Hospital staff's efforts to provide for your needs after you left the hospital

❏ ❏ ❏ ❏ ❏ ❏

BILLING BY HOSPITAL

51. EXPLANATIONS ABOUT COSTS AND HOW TO HANDLE YOUR HOSPITAL BILLS: The completeness and accuracy of information and the willingness of hospital staff to answer your questions about finances

❏ ❏ ❏ ❏ ❏ ❏

52. EFFICIENCY OF BILLING: How fast you got your bill, how accurate and understandable it was

❏ ❏ ❏ ❏ ❏ ❏

LOOKING BACK ON YOUR CARE

53. HOSPITAL QUALITY: Overall quality of care and services you received from the hospital

❏ ❏ ❏ ❏ ❏ ❏

54. THE OUTCOME OF YOUR HOSPITAL STAY: How much you were helped by the hospitalization

❏ ❏ ❏ ❏ ❏ ❏

55. HOSPITAL IMAGE: How good the hospital's reputation is in your community

❏ ❏ ❏ ❏ ❏ ❏

OVERALL SATISFACTION WITH HOSPITAL

Here are things that people sometimes say about their hospital stay. Please tell us whether you *strongly agree, somewhat agree, somewhat disagree,* or *strongly disagree* with each statement.

	Strongly agree	Somewhat agree	Somewhat disagree	Strongly disagree
56. The care I received at the hospital was so good that I have bragged about it to family and friends.	❏	❏	❏	❏
57. At all times it was clear to me which doctor was responsible for my care.	❏	❏	❏	❏

RECOMMENDATIONS AND SUGGESTIONS

58. Would you recommend this hospital to your family and friends if they needed hospital care?

❏ 1 Definitely would
❏ 2 Probably would
❏ 3 Probably would not

❏ 4 Definitely would not
❏ 5 Does not apply to me because I do not live near hospital

59. How likely would you be to return to this hospital if you ever need to be hospitalized again?

❏ 1 I'm 100% sure that I'd return
❏ 2 It's very likely that I'd return
❏ 3 I probably would return
❏ 4 I'm not sure if I would return
❏ 5 I probably would not return

❏ 6 It's very unlikely that I'd return
❏ 7 I'm 100% sure that I would not return
❏ 8 Does not apply to me because I do not live near hospital

60. Why would you return or not return to this hospital? Please give us your honest opinions. Also, if you would not return, where would you rather go and why?

_____
_____
_____
_____
_____
_____

61. NEEDED IMPROVEMENTS: Please tell us what the hospital could do to improve the quality of the care and services that you received and do a better job of meeting your needs.

_____
_____
_____
_____
_____
_____
_____
_____
_____

62. GOOD OR BAD SURPRISES: Did anything happen during your stay in the hospital that surprised you? If so, please tell us what it was.

GOOD SURPRISES:_____

_____
_____
_____
_____

BAD SURPRISES:_____

_____
_____
_____
_____

If you need additional space for comments feel free to attach additional pages.

FACTS ABOUT YOU

These next few questions are for statistical purposes.

63. What was the last grade of school you (the patient) completed?

❑ 1 Eighth grade or less
❑ 2 Some high school
❑ 3 High school graduate
❑ 4 Technical/Trade/Vocational school (after high school)
❑ 5 Some college
❑ 6 Two-year college graduate
❑ 7 Four-year college graduate
❑ 8 Postgraduate

64. You are . . .

❑ 1 White
❑ 2 Black
❑ 3 Hispanic
❑ 4 Oriental
❑ 5 American Indian
❑ 6 Other (Specify):_____

65. In the past six months, where have you heard, seen or read anything about this hospital? ("X" all that apply.)

❑ 1 Family or friends
❑ 2 From a doctor
❑ 3 From other medical persons or hospital employees
❑ 4 Through my work
❑ 5 Television
❑ 6 Newspaper
❑ 7 Radio
❑ 8 Magazines
❑ 9 Billboards
❑ 10 Printed material through the mail
❑ 11 Other ways (Specify)_____

66. Have you received your bill(s) from the hospital?

❑ 1 Yes, it came in less than two weeks
❑ 2 Yes, it came in two to four weeks
❑ 3 Yes, it took more than four weeks
❑ 4 No, I have not yet received my bill
❑ 5 Does not apply to me

67. What type of health insurance, if any, do you expect to pay for most of your hospital bill? ("X" all that apply.)

❑ 1 None
❑ 2 Blue Cross/Blue Shield
❑ 3 Medicare
❑ 4 Medicaid
❑ 5 Other type of government program
❑ 6 Private or commercial health insurance plan (e.g. Prudential, Aetna)
❑ 7 Health Maintenance Organization (HMO) or other plan which names the hospital or physician you must (Specify)_____
❑ 8 Other insurance (Specify)_____
❑ 9 I don't know the type of insurance

68. From time to time, we wish to telephone people to ask a few more questions that are raised by a patient's answers. Please "X" the box below and include your phone number if you give permission to contact you should the need arise.

❑ Yes, My phone number is:
(_____)_____
Area Code

Thank you for your time and assistance!

Please double check to make sure you answered all questions. Then mail the questionnaire in the postage-paid envelope to: NCG Research, 2100 West End Avenue, Suite 800, Nashville, TN 37203.

Department Specific Patient Satisfaction Survey

Critical Care Patient Satisfaction Survey

Dear Patients and Families:
We are concerned about your opinions regarding the care you or your loved one received in the *critical care unit*. Your feedback will help us to evaluate and identify areas in which we can improve our nursing care. Your time and thoughtful consideration in answering this survey is greatly appreciated. Additional written comments are most welcome. We would like to hear from both patients and family members whenever possible. We invite family members to help patients complete this survey if needed. Please be assured that your responses will remain anonymous. Thank you for your assistance.

OVERALL SATISFACTION

1. Who is completing this survey?
❏ Patient   ❏ Family member   ❏ Other (please specify) _____

2. Critical care unit the patient was admitted to: (Check all that apply.)
❏ CVICU   ❏ MICU   ❏ SICU   ❏ Burn Unit

3. How long did the patient spend in this unit?
❏ 3 days or less   ❏ 4 to 8 days   ❏ 9 to 14 days   ❏ 15 days or more

4. Are you currently:
❏ Hospitalized   ❏ Discharged
   If you are still hospitalized, are you in the critical care unit or general nursing unit?_____

5. What did you like BEST about your experience in the critical care unit?_____
_____
_____

6. What did you like LEAST about your experience in the critical care unit?_____
_____

NURSING CARE

For the following questions, mark the appropriate space that best describes your *critical care* experience. Concentrate on the capitalized, key words of each question. Please skip any item that does not apply to your experience.

7. The ORIENTATION TO THE UNIT was

❏ Excellent ❏ Good ❏ Satisfactory ❏ Fair ❏ Poor

8. The UNIT HANDBOOK was

❏ Excellent ❏ Good ❏ Satisfactory ❏ Fair ❏ Poor

9. The FLEXIBILITY OF VISITING HOURS was

❏ Excellent ❏ Good ❏ Satisfactory ❏ Fair ❏ Poor

10. The WAITING ROOM FACILITIES were

❏ Excellent ❏ Good ❏ Satisfactory ❏ Fair ❏ Poor

11. The FAMILY SUPPORT GROUP MEETING in the unit was

❏ Excellent ❏ Good ❏ Satisfactory ❏ Fair ❏ Poor

12. The way the nurses SHOWED CONCERN AND COMPASSION was

❏ Excellent ❏ Good ❏ Satisfactory ❏ Fair ❏ Poor

13. The way the nurses TOOK TIME to explain things to me was

❏ Excellent ❏ Good ❏ Satisfactory ❏ Fair ❏ Poor

14. The way the nurses LISTENED TO ME was

❏ Excellent ❏ Good ❏ Satisfactory ❏ Fair ❏ Poor

15. The PATIENCE of the nurses who cared for me was

❏ Excellent ❏ Good ❏ Satisfactory ❏ Fair ❏ Poor

16. The CARING ATTITUDE of the nurses was

❏ Excellent ❏ Good ❏ Satisfactory ❏ Fair ❏ Poor

17. OVERALL, the PERSONAL CHARACTERISTICS of the nurses were

❏ Excellent ❏ Good ❏ Satisfactory ❏ Fair ❏ Poor

18. The way the nurses were THERE FOR ME WHEN NEEDED was

❏ Excellent ❏ Good ❏ Satisfactory ❏ Fair ❏ Poor

19. The way the nurses PERSONALIZED my care to meet MY NEEDS was

❏ Excellent ❏ Good ❏ Satisfactory ❏ Fair ❏ Poor

20. The way the nurses WATCHED OVER ME was

❑ Excellent ❑ Good ❑ Satisfactory ❑ Fair ❑ Poor

21. The information from the nurses about what I could do TO HELP MYSELF while in the critical care unit was

❑ Excellent ❑ Good ❑ Satisfactory ❑ Fair ❑ Poor

22. The suggestions from nurses on the ALTERNATIVES or OPTIONS for my care were

❑ Excellent ❑ Good ❑ Satisfactory ❑ Fair ❑ Poor

23. The suggestions from nurses on how to DEAL WITH MY STRESS were

❑ Excellent ❑ Good ❑ Satisfactory ❑ Fair ❑ Poor

24. The explanations/teaching the nurses provided on my condition, tests, procedures, and treatments were at a LEVEL I COULD UNDERSTAND

❑ Excellent ❑ Good ❑ Satisfactory ❑ Fair ❑ Poor

25. The suggestions from the nurses about OTHER HOSPITAL PER-SONNEL who could help me with SPECIAL PROBLEMS were

❑ Excellent ❑ Good ❑ Satisfactory ❑ Fair ❑ Poor

26. The way the nurses on all the shifts WORKED TOGETHER ON MY CARE was

❑ Excellent ❑ Good ❑ Satisfactory ❑ Fair ❑ Poor

27. The information SHARED WITH MY FAMILY by the nursing staff was

❑ Excellent ❑ Good ❑ Satisfactory ❑ Fair ❑ Poor

28. The way the nurses attempted to UNDERSTAND MY SITUATION was

❑ Excellent ❑ Good ❑ Satisfactory ❑ Fair ❑ Poor

29. The AVAILABILITY of nurses to meet family needs during and between visiting hours was

❑ Excellent ❑ Good ❑ Satisfactory ❑ Fair ❑ Poor

30. The PRIVATE TIME the nurses gave us during visiting hours was

❑ Excellent ❑ Good ❑ Satisfactory ❑ Fair ❑ Poor

31. The encouragement of nurses about how the family could HELP THE PATIENT (feeding, bathing, emotional support) was

❑ Excellent ❑ Good ❑ Satisfactory ❑ Fair ❑ Poor

32. The SUPPORT provided by the nurses at the bedside during stressful times (procedures, visiting hours) was

❑ Excellent ❑ Good ❑ Satisfactory ❑ Fair ❑ Poor

33. The AMOUNT OF TIME the nurses spent with me was

❑ Excellent ❑ Good ❑ Satisfactory ❑ Fair ❑ Poor

34. The way the nurses were COMFORTABLE in answering my questions was

❑ Excellent ❑ Good ❑ Satisfactory ❑ Fair ❑ Poor

35. The way the nurses INVOLVED the family in MAKING DECISIONS about the patient's care was

❑ Excellent ❑ Good ❑ Satisfactory ❑ Fair ❑ Poor

36. The way the nurses REPEATED INFORMATION in DIFFERENT FORMS (conversations/booklets) was

❑ Excellent ❑ Good ❑ Satisfactory ❑ Fair ❑ Poor

37. The TIMELINESS OF INFORMATION provided by the nurses about the patient's condition and treatment was

❑ Excellent ❑ Good ❑ Satisfactory ❑ Fair ❑ Poor

38. The way the HEALTH CARE TEAM COMMUNICATED with us was

❑ Excellent ❑ Good ❑ Satisfactory ❑ Fair ❑ Poor

39. The way the nursing staff controlled UNNECESSARY NOISE was

❑ Excellent ❑ Good ❑ Satisfactory ❑ Fair ❑ Poor

40. The way the nurses responded to my needs for PAIN MANAGEMENT was

❑ Excellent ❑ Good ❑ Satisfactory ❑ Fair ❑ Poor

41. The PROFICIENCY of the nurses in the TECHNICAL ASPECTS of my care was

❑ Excellent ❑ Good ❑ Satisfactory ❑ Fair ❑ Poor

42. PREPARATION FOR TRANSFER to another unit was

❑ Excellent ❑ Good ❑ Satisfactory ❑ Fair ❑ Poor

43. Overall, HOW SATISFIED were you with the care you received in this critical care unit?

❑ Excellent ❑ Good ❑ Satisfactory ❑ Fair ❑ Poor

Feel free to add any additional comments (please also mention any nurses you considered to be outstanding). Please use additional sheet if desired.

_____
_____
_____
_____
_____
_____

GENERAL INFORMATION

Please answer the following questions related to your personal characteristics:

Age _____

Male or female _____

Number of times hospitalized at UIHC as an adult _____

OPTIONAL

Name   _____

Address   _____

            _____

            _____

Phone   _____

Thank you for your help. We appreciate the time you took in sharing your thoughts.

SOURCE: Created by the authors based on a survey originally developed by Mary Beth Petersen, Director of Hospital Education, St Michael Hospital, Milwaukee, WI, originally published in Rowland HS, and Rowland BL: _The Manual of Nursing Quality Assurance_, vol 1, exhibit 27–3. Gaithersburg, MD: Aspen Publishers, Inc, 1987.

Index

satisfaction surveys and, 52. *See also* Satisfaction surveys
systematic method for, 31
See also specific methods
Data management, *AMH* and, 112
Decision aid, 81
Decision makers
  Joint Commission standards and patient's family as, 12
  patients as, 17, 81
Designing work processes, 6, 7, 32, 62
  "key quality characteristics" and, 64, 65
  AMH and, 114
  in cycle for improving performance, 33, 35, 36
  example of, 63
  patient input in, 10, 12, 14, 36-43
    goal in, 64
    steps in using, 70-74
    "voice of the customer" table for, 100
  and reducing/eliminating variations, 119
  successful, 64, 65, 74
  See also Redesigning work processes
"Design specifications," 64
DHMC. *See* Dartmouth-Hitchcock Medical Center (DHMC)
Diagnosis
  communication failure and problems with, 19
  measurement method according to type of, 44
  patient groups according to, 37
Diagnosis related groups (DRGs), 80
Direct observation, 47, 48, 49
  needs assessment and, 51
  satisfaction surveys and, 52
Discharge checklist for patient, 57
Discussion group, 81
DRGs. *See* Diagnosis related groups (DRGs)

Education
  of nurses, 84, 86
  of patients, 17, 23, 72
    example of (patient information for breast cancer), 81-82
    example of (reengineering for patient-centered care), 86, 89
  of staff
    AMH and, 112
    regarding patient participation, 96
  See also Training
Effectiveness, 38, 40, 71
  AMH and, 108, 110
  example of (pain management), 83
  listed on matrix for patient input, 73
  measurement and, 33
Efficacy, 38, 40, 71
  AMH and, 108, 110
  listed on matrix for patient input, 73
Efficiency, 38, 40, 71
  AMH and, 108, 110
  example of (reengineering for patient-centered care), 85, 86, 93

Physicians
  as "customers," 26-29, 93, 94
  expectations of patients vs., 96
  extra patient time with, 22
  information for, 93
  interpersonal skills of, 15, 19
  listening to, 27, 29
  pain management and, 83
  patients' relationships with, 15, 19
  patients' understanding of instructions from, 11
  and patients as "customers," 5-6, 25
  perceptions of patients vs., 42
  referring, 93, 94, 98-104
Picker Institute, 86, 88
Plan-Do-Check-Act (PDCA) cycle, 7, 54, 95. *See also* Plan-Do-Study-Act (PDSA) cycle
Plan-Do-Study-Act (PDSA) cycle, 66, 67
Planning, 35, 54, 66
  AMH and, 113-114, 120
  design and, 114
  quality function deployment and, 97, 98
  sample form for, 45-46
Population, in measurement for patient input, 46, 50
Practice guidelines. *See* Clinical practice guidelines
Priorities of patients, 6, 97, 101
  and organizational priority setting, 35
Priority setting, 6-7
  AMH and, 111, 120
  assessment and, 57
  in cycle for improving performance, 33, 35, 36
  example of (quality function deployment), 97, 101, 102
  in gathering patient input, 22, 43
  listening and, 28
  in measuring, 22
Process analysis, 6
Processes
  affecting key functions. *See* Functions
  AMH and, 111, 115
  assessment of, 35
  in cycle for improving performance, 33, 34
  data collection about, 34
  defined in *AMH*, 107, 113
  high-risk, 34, 43
  high-volume, 34, 43
  indicators and, 51
  measurement method according to type of, 44
  opportunities for improvement and, 109
  over time, 117, 118
  patient input and, 64, 71-74
  problem-prone, 34, 35, 43, 109, 116
  "real-time" measurement of, 56
  related to important functions, 34, 36, 37-92, 116
  See also Work processes
"Process requirements," 64
Product needs, patient needs/expectations regarding, 16
"Product requirements," 64

QFD. *See* Quality function deployment (QFD)
Qualitative data, 49, 58
  assessment of, 58
  quality function deployment and, 101
Quality assurance,"take-it-for-granted" attributes and, 20
Quality control, *AMH* and, 117
"Quality cube," 41
Quality function deployment (QFD), 70-71
  example of (quality function deployment), 93-104
  first use of, 96
  steps in, 97-103
Quality improvement, 62-74
  "coach" for, 28
  four examples of, 77-106
  intensive efforts in, 43, 62
  list of articles and books on, 124-125
  patient input and, 12-13, 24-26
  patients' perspective and, 24-26
  tools for, 66-74
Quality-of-life measures, 109
Quantitative data, 49, 51, 59, 62
  assessment of, 59, 62
  quality function deployment and, 101
Questionnaire, 28. *See also* Surveys
Questions
  follow-up, 50
  open-ended, 49, 54

"Real-time" measurement, 56-57
Redesigning work processes, 7, 62, 64
  "key quality characteristics" and, 64, 65
  in cycle for improving performance, 33, 35, 36
  example of (pain management), 82-85
  for "exciting attributes," 24
  to give patients more information, 64
  patient input and, 10, 72-74, 100
  successful, 64, 65, 74
Reference databases, 9, 109, 113, 114, 118
Referring physicians, 93, 94, 98-104
Relevance, 113, 115, 116, 119
  and designing work processes, 120
Reliability, 23, 43
  indicators and, 51
Research
  list of articles and books on, 123-126
  methods, 46, 47, 72
Resources, 28-29
  AMH and, 112, 120
  and designing work processes, 32
  human
    AMH and, 112, 121
    and patient needs for information, 80-81
  list of articles and books as, 123-126
  measurement and, 33, 53

UMMC. *See* University of Michigan Medical Center (UMMC)
University of Chicago Hospitals, 85-93
University of Michigan Medical Center (UMMC), 93-104
University of Wisconsin Hospitals (UWH), 78-82
Utilization-management activities, 116
Utilization review, 54

"Value compass," 55-56
Variance, 113
Variation, 59, 62, 113, 117
  designing work processes to reduce/eliminate, 119
  intensive assessment and, 118-119
Vendors, 29. *See also* Suppliers
Videos, interactive, 17-18
Vision, 55
  AMH and, 114
  and designing work processes, 32, 37
  priority setting and, 43
Visitors, accommodation of, 20
"Voice of the customer," 96-100. *See also* Listening

Waiting times (for patients), 60-62, 64, 93
Work processes, 6, 32-34
  cycle for improvement in, 31-76
  designing. *See* Designing work processes
  See also Performance